FRAILTY AND NUTRITION

Powering Resilience

Dr Saifuddin Ekram

ISBN-13: 979-8305444049
Independently Published

Cover design by: Art Painter

Printed in the United States of America

To my daughter, Synthia, with love and appreciation~

CONTENTS

Title Page

Copyright

Dedication

Introduction

Chapter 1: Understanding Frailty ... 1

Chapter 2: Role of Nutrition in Frailty ... 10

Chapter 3: Macronutrients and Frailty ... 23

Chapter 4: Micronutrients and Frailty ... 31

Chapter 5: Malnutrition and Frailty ... 41

Chapter 6: Gut and Frailty Link ... 53

Chapter 7: Practical Nutrition Strategies for Frail Adults ... 61

Chapter 8: Future of Nutrition and Frailty Research ... 70

Abbreviations ... 76

References ... 78

INTRODUCTION

Aging is an intricate journey—a path filled with wisdom, reflection, and, at times, challenges to health and independence. Among these challenges lies frailty, a condition that silently chips away at an individual's strength, resilience, and ability to bounce back from physical, cognitive or emotional stress. Yet, frailty is not an inevitable consequence of aging. Increasingly, science is revealing its modifiable nature, with nutrition emerging as one of the most promising tools to combat frailty and foster vitality. This book, 'Frailty and Nutrition: Powering Resilience', explores this critical connection, providing insights, strategies, and hope for older adults, caregivers, and healthcare professionals alike.

Frailty isn't just about physical weakness—it's a multifaceted condition that intertwines the physical, cognitive, and social dimensions of health. It affects how individuals move, think, and interact with the world around them, placing them at a higher risk of multiple adverse health events like falls, hospitalizations, and reduced quality of life. But at its heart lies a fascinating interplay of factors, many of which can be influenced by something as basic as what we eat. Nutrition holds the power to strengthen bones, maintain muscles, sharpen minds, and fortify the immune system, offering a path to resilience even in the face of aging.

This book takes you on a journey through the complex relationship between frailty and nutrition. It begins by explaining frailty, exploring its prevalence, risk factors, and the various ways it manifests in physical, mental, and social domains. Early identification and timely intervention are emphasized as key steps in preventing frailty from advancing to more serious health challenges.

The role of nutrition is then explored in depth, presenting it as a factor that can significantly influence frailty. The foods we consume, or fail to consume, can either weaken or strengthen our capacity to cope with aging. This includes understanding the contributions of both macronutrients, such as protein, carbohydrates, and fats, and micronutrients, like vitamins, minerals, and antioxidants. Each nutrient plays a unique role in supporting muscle strength, energy balance, cognitive function, and overall resilience.

The complex relationship between malnutrition and frailty is a recurring theme, as the two often coexist and worsen each other. This book highlights practical ways to identify and address malnutrition, offering tools and strategies that empower individuals and caregivers to break this cycle. It also delves into the fascinating connection between gut health and frailty, shedding light on how a healthy microbiome can support resilience and overall well-being.

For those seeking practical guidance in an easy and simple language, this book offers actionable advice on meal planning, nutritional supplementation, overcoming appetite challenges, and creating affordable, culturally sensitive dietary solutions. Finally, it looks to the future, showcasing innovations in personalized nutrition, technological advancements, and public health policies that hold promise for combating frailty through nutrition.

Frailty is not destiny. With the right knowledge and strategies, it is possible to age with strength, dignity, and vitality. Let this book guide you in harnessing the power of nutrition to embrace resilience and thrive at every stage of life.

CHAPTER 1: UNDERSTANDING FRAILTY

Frailty is a condition that captures the interplay of aging, health, and resilience. Imagine your body as a ship. Over time, wear and tear happen; a frail ship is one that, even with a small wave, might tip precariously. Let us set sail into the details of frailty and why understanding it matters so much.

1.1 Definition And Key Characteristics Of Frailty

Frailty is not just about feeling weak or perpetually tired; it is a deeper, more complex condition. Imagine the body's systems as a team—when everyone is at peak performance, you are unstoppable. But with frailty, the players (your organs, muscles, and brain) are worn out, slow, or simply not showing up for the game. Even the smallest hiccup—a cold, a skipped meal, or a bad night's sleep—can lead to a cascade of complications.

Medically speaking, frailty is defined as a state of increased vulnerability. This vulnerability comes from a decline across multiple physiological systems, leaving the body unable to recover easily from stress. Think of it like a smartphone with too many apps running in the background—the battery drains faster, and a simple task, like opening another app, can cause the whole system to crash.

The Key Characteristics

Fried Frailty Phenotype: One of the most widely accepted frameworks to define frailty comes from the research of Dr. Linda Fried and colleagues (1). They identified five hallmark indicators that can help detect frailty:

Unintentional Weight Loss: Losing more than 4.5 kg (about 10 pounds) in a year without trying is a red flag. It is not about fitting into old jeans; it is a signal that the body's energy reserves are dwindling.

Exhaustion: This is not your average "I've had a long day" tiredness. It is a deep, persistent fatigue that does not improve with rest.

Weak Grip Strength: If a handshake feels more like a limp fish than a confident squeeze, it could indicate muscle decline.

Slow Walking Speed: Walking becomes less of a stride and more of a shuffle, a sign that mobility and coordination are waning.

Low Physical Activity: When gardening, shopping, or even climbing stairs feels like climbing Mount Everest, it is time to pay attention.

Other Frameworks of Frailty

Frailty Index: The Frailty Index (FI) is a tool used to measure the health status of older individuals. It was developed by Dr. Kenneth Rockwood and Dr. Arnold Mitnitski at Dalhousie University in Canada (2, 3). The FI is calculated by dividing the number of health deficits present in an individual by the total number of age-related health variables considered. This index serves as a proxy measure of aging and vulnerability to poor outcomes.

Clinical Frailty Scale (CFS): This is a seven-point scale ranging from very fit to severely frail. It provides a single descriptor of a person's level of frailty based on clinical judgment (4).

Edmonton Frail Scale (EFS): This scale evaluates frailty based on nine components, including cognition, general health, functional independence, social support, medication use, nutrition, mood, continence, and functional performance. It categorizes individuals into five levels of frailty from not frail to severe frailty (5).

FRAIL Scale: This is a five-item questionnaire assessing **F**atigue, **R**esistance, **A**mbulation, **I**llnesses, and **L**oss of weight. It is used to screen for frailty in clinical settings (5).

There are many approaches to assessing frailty. Each method provides a unique view on frailty, enabling healthcare providers to customize their evaluations and interventions based on individual requirements.

Frailty in Everyday Terms

Think of frailty as the body's diminishing ability to bounce back. Remember when you were younger, and a bad flu would knock you down for a couple of days? You would bounce back after some chicken soup and sleep. For someone who is frail, that same flu can lead to a spiral of hospital visits, immobility, and even long-term disability. It is like a Jenga tower that has been played for hours—remove one more block, and the whole structure could collapse.

Frailty also comes with what experts call "unstable disability," meaning day-to-day abilities fluctuate wildly. One day, an individual might manage to dress independently, and the next, they struggle with basic tasks. This unpredictability makes frailty even harder to cope with—for both the individual and their caregivers.

Why It Matters

Frailty is not just about the person experiencing it; it is a societal challenge. As populations age and people live longer, frailty is becoming more common. Research shows that frailty rates differ widely among different populations. Women tend to experience higher rates of frailty than men, and the likelihood of being frail increases with age (6). Frailty also places a significant burden on healthcare systems, leading to higher costs due to more frequent hospital visits and longer recovery periods (7). Additionally, frailty rates vary by region, influenced by local healthcare systems, lifestyles, and socioeconomic conditions (6). Addressing frailty requires targeted strategies tailored to the specific needs of each region to improve the quality of life for older adults and manage healthcare costs effectively.

Imagine a world where frailty is better understood and managed. Healthcare providers could tailor treatments to focus on what truly matters to individuals. Communities could develop programs that keep older adults engaged and active. Families could recognize the early signs of frailty and act before it leads to more significant health issues.

Let us lighten things up a bit: if frailty were a person, it would be that grouchy neighbour who is always saying, "One wrong move, and it is all downhill from here!" But instead of avoiding them, we need to get to know them better. Why? Because understanding frailty helps us prepare for it, prevent it when possible, and manage it effectively when it is unavoidable.

The good news? Frailty does not have to be a foregone conclusion. By recognizing its early signs and understanding its key characteristics, we can take steps to intervene. Exercise, proper nutrition, and staying socially connected are just a few of the tools we will explore in the next sections. After all, the more we know about frailty, the better we can navigate aging with resilience and grace.

1.2 Prevalence And Risk Factors In Older Adults

Frailty becomes more common as we age. Here are some recent findings:

Global Prevalence: A study looking at data from 62 countries found that frailty rates vary a lot. About 12% of people aged 50 and older are frail based on physical measures. When using a different method (frailty index), this number goes up to 24%. Pre-frailty, a stage before full frailty, affects 46% using physical measures and 49% using the frailty index (6).

Gender Differences: Frailty is more common in women than men. Using physical measures,

15% of women are frail compared to 11% of men. With the frailty index, 29% of women are frail compared to 20% of men (6).

Age-Related Increase: Frailty rates go up with age. Older age groups have higher rates, so early detection and intervention are crucial (6).

Economic Impact: For example, in Australia, frailty places a heavy burden on the healthcare system. Frail older adults have higher healthcare costs due to more frequent hospital visits and longer recovery times. Over three years, healthcare costs for frail individuals were estimated at $1.28 billion, compared to $885 million for non-frail individuals (7).

Regional Variations: Frailty rates differ between countries and regions, influenced by healthcare systems, lifestyles, and socioeconomic conditions. This means we need strategies tailored to different regions to address frailty effectively (6).

These findings highlight the need to address frailty with targeted healthcare strategies to improve the quality of life for older adults and reduce healthcare costs. With these statistics in mind, understanding frailty is crucial for planning healthcare and community resources.

What does this mean in everyday terms? It is like walking into a room of centenarians and realizing that half of them might struggle with simple tasks like climbing stairs or getting out of bed.

Risk Factors

Frailty can affect anyone, but some risk factors make it more likely to show up uninvited. Let us break them down:

Age: While frailty is not a guaranteed consequence of getting older, the odds increase significantly with each passing year. It is like wrinkles; not everyone gets them early, but they are more common with time.

Lifestyle Choices: Sedentary habits, poor nutrition, and smoking act as sneaky saboteurs. Think of your body as a garden: without care, weeds (like inactivity) take over, and the soil (your health) erodes.

Social Isolation: Humans are wired for connection. Loneliness is not just an emotional burden—it can literally wear down the body's defences. Being socially isolated is like operating a smartphone in airplane mode: functional, but not thriving.

Chronic Diseases: Conditions like diabetes mellitus, heart disease, and arthritis chip away at resilience. Imagine carrying a backpack filled with bricks; each illness adds weight, making it harder to stay upright.

A Mixed Bag

Here is where it gets intriguing: frailty is not an inevitability. Some nonagenarians are out there playing tennis, while others in their sixties might struggle to walk a block. Why? It is a mix of genetics, environment, and life choices. You might inherit good genes, but if you treat your body like a clunker, it will run like one.

Think of aging bodies as cars. Some vintage models from the 1970s still zip around with ease because their owners have been meticulous with maintenance—frequent oil changes (healthy diet), tire rotations (exercise), and careful driving (avoiding smoking and stress). Meanwhile, some newer cars sputter and stall, victims of neglect and hard use. The lesson? Whether you are a Cadillac or a Corolla, upkeep matters!

Why These Numbers Matter

The sobering statistics around frailty serve as a wake-up call. As lifespans increase, so does the need to focus on healthspan—the years of life spent in good health. If half of the over-85 population faces frailty, then the healthcare system, communities, and families need to be prepared to offer support. But more importantly, interventions can be implemented earlier to keep frailty at bay.

Prevention: The Silver Lining

Here is the hopeful part: frailty is not destiny. Engaging in regular physical activity, eating balanced meals rich in nutrients, staying socially connected, and managing chronic diseases can significantly reduce the risk. Think of these habits as adding reinforcements to that metaphorical Jenga tower, making it sturdier and less likely to topple with a small nudge.

Frailty does not have to define your later years. By understanding its prevalence and risk factors, you can chart a course toward resilience and vitality. After all, age is just a number; how you live it makes all the difference.

1.3 Physical, Cognitive, And Social Dimensions Of Frailty

Frailty is not just about muscles; it is a three-ring circus of physical, cognitive, and social aspects. Each dimension can affect the others, creating a feedback loop that can make managing frailty quite a challenge. Let us explore each ring of this circus in detail.

Physical: The Muscle Meltdown

The Physical Dimension of Frailty: When we talk about the physical dimension of frailty, we are referring to the tangible, sometimes stubborn aspects of our bodies that can show signs of wear and tear. One of the biggest causes here is sarcopenia—a term used for muscle loss. It is a natural part of aging but can be accelerated by inactivity and poor nutrition.

Loss of Strength: Loss of muscle strength is one of the first hints of frailty. Remember when you could carry all the groceries in one trip without breaking a sweat? Now, those same bags feel like they are filled with lead. This reduction in strength can make daily tasks, such as climbing stairs or lifting a kettle, seem like major undertakings.

Balance Issues: Balance, or the lack thereof, also plays a big role in physical frailty. As we age, our muscles and joints do not respond as quickly, leading to a higher risk of falls. These balance issues are often due to a combination of weaker muscles, slower reflexes, and changes in our vision and inner ear function.

Fatigue: Fatigue is another key player. It is not just about feeling tired after a long day; it is about an overwhelming sense of exhaustion that does not go away with rest. This continuing fatigue can make even the simplest activities feel like climbing Everest. It is like your body's "low battery" warning is stuck on, no matter how much you try to recharge.

Cognitive: The Brainy Brouhaha

Cognitive frailty is the mental equivalent of misplacing your keys—everywhere. It includes memory lapses, slower thinking, and in severe cases, conditions like Alzheimer's. Cognitive decline can start subtly and progress over time, affecting everything from problem-solving skills to language and decision-making.

Memory Lapses: We all forget things from time to time, but frequent memory lapses can be a sign of cognitive frailty. It might start with forgetting where you put your glasses, but over time, it can lead to missing important appointments or struggling to remember the names of close friends and family.

Slower Thinking: Ever feel like your brain is moving in slow motion? Cognitive frailty often includes a noticeable slowdown in thinking processes. It can take longer to process information, make decisions, or follow conversations. It is like your mind is buffering, but the progress bar never quite reaches 100%.

Cognitive Conditions: Conditions like Alzheimer's and other forms of dementia are more common in individuals with cognitive frailty. These conditions not only affect memory but can also change personality, behavior, and the ability to perform everyday tasks.

Social: The Overlooked Ringmaster

Social frailty is like the ringmaster of this three-ring circus—often overlooked but critically important. Social connections play a huge role in our overall well-being. Isolation, widowhood, or living far from family can amplify the effects of physical and cognitive frailty.

Isolation: Social isolation can happen for many reasons—mobility issues, the loss of loved ones, or even retiring from work. When you are not engaging with others regularly, it can lead to feelings of loneliness and depression. This isolation can, in turn, worsen cognitive decline and physical health.

Widowhood: Losing a spouse or partner is a profound experience that can accelerate frailty. The emotional impact can be overwhelming, and without a strong social network, it is easy to become isolated and disconnected. This can lead to a downward spiral of declining health.

Living Far from Family: Living far from family can mean less support and fewer opportunities for social interaction. While technology can help bridge the gap, it is not the same as having loved ones nearby. This lack of close social ties can make it harder to cope with the challenges of frailty.

How They Interconnect: The Domino Effect

Picture frailty as a domino effect. Each dimension does not exist in isolation; they are all interconnected. A fall (physical) can lead to a fear of leaving the house (social), which can, in turn, worsen mental sharpness (cognitive). This domino effect means that addressing one dimension can have positive effects on the others.

The Physical-Social Connection: For example, improving physical strength through exercise can boost confidence and reduce the risk of falls. This increased confidence can encourage more social interaction, which can have positive effects on mental health.

The Cognitive-Social Connection: Engaging in social activities can help keep the mind sharp. Interacting with others, solving problems, and engaging in conversations are all great ways to stimulate cognitive function.

The Physical-Cognitive Connection: Physical exercise also benefits the brain. Activities that get the heart pumping can improve blood flow to the brain, enhancing cognitive function and reducing the risk of cognitive decline.

So, frailty is a complex, multi-dimensional issue that requires a holistic approach. By understanding the physical, cognitive, and social dimensions, we can better address the challenges and improve the quality of life for those affected. Remember, tackling one dimension can benefit the others, creating a positive feedback loop that helps manage frailty more effectively.

1.4 Importance Of Early Identification And Intervention

Here is the good news: frailty is not a one-way street. Spotting it early can change the game, transforming potential decline into an opportunity for proactive action.

Clues to Watch

Recognizing the early markers of frailty is like being a detective with a keen eye for clues. Here are some telltale indicators that should not be ignored:

Slower Walking Speed: If your brisk morning walk has turned into a slow shuffle, it is worth noting. This is not just a quirk of aging; it is a signal your body might need some attention.

Struggling with Basic Activities: Tasks like dressing, bathing, or even opening a jar should not feel like a gym workout. If they do, it is a red flag.

Persistent Fatigue: Feeling unusually tired most of the time? Take note. This is not about needing an extra cup of coffee; it is about your body's energy reserves being perpetually low.

These are not just quirks of getting older—they are calls to action, nudging you to pay attention and take steps before these issues escalate.

Interventions

Taking action early can make a significant difference. Here are some effective strategies to manage and mitigate frailty:

Exercise: Strength training is not just for bodybuilders. Even light resistance exercises can help frail individuals regain muscle and confidence (8). Think of it as your body's own version of a tune-up.

Nutrition: A diet rich in protein, vitamin D, and omega-3 fatty acids can combat frailty (9). It is like giving your body the premium fuel it needs to function at its best.

Social Engagement: Never underestimate the power of a regular coffee date or a community class. Social interactions are not just fun—they are protective, boosting your mental and emotional well-being (10).

Medical Care: Comprehensive geriatric assessments can tailor treatments to individual needs, ensuring that every aspect of your health is considered (11). It is like having a personalized roadmap to better health.

Why Early is Better

Think of frailty like a crack in a windshield. Ignore it, and it spreads, turning into a web of issues that can be much harder to fix. Spot it early, and you can address it before it becomes a bigger problem. Early intervention allows for more effective management and can prevent the rapid progression of frailty, keeping you healthier and more active for longer.

Wrapping It Up

Frailty might sound intimidating, but understanding it empowers us. Whether you are reading this for yourself or a loved one, remember: knowledge is the first step in staying resilient. With the right strategies, that ship can keep sailing steady, no matter how choppy the waters get. Taking steps to address frailty early ensures that you or your loved ones can continue to enjoy life's journey with strength and vitality.

CHAPTER 2: ROLE OF NUTRITION IN FRAILTY

Frailty does not strike like lightning from a clear sky; it is more like a slow drizzle eroding the foundation of a building over time. This phenomenon stems from a complex interplay of factors—aging, genetics, lifestyle choices, chronic diseases, and, notably, nutrition. Yet, where there is rain, there is also a chance for rainbows. Nutrition, a modifiable risk factor, stands out as a bright beacon of hope in the frailty narrative. By exploring its nuances and connections to frailty, we unlock a powerful tool to foster resilience in older adults. Let us dive into the symphony that nutrition orchestrates within the body.

2.1 How Nutrition Impacts Frailty

Imagine your body as a finely tuned orchestra, where every instrument must play in harmony to perform a masterpiece. In this metaphor, nutrition is the conductor. When the conductor leads well, the symphony thrives. But when it falters, the performance falls apart. Frailty, then, is akin to a cacophony—a loss of coordination among vital processes like muscle strength, immune function, and energy regulation (12).

The Protective Armor of Good Nutrition

Scientific evidence showcases the profound impact of diet quality on frailty risk (13). Think of fruits, vegetables, and whole grains as the superheroes of the nutritional world, donning their antioxidant capes and anti-inflammatory shields. These foods reduce oxidative stress and inflammation—two villains in the frailty saga. Guess what? Your dinner plate could be your secret weapon against frailty as you age. Research says that high-quality diets like the Mediterranean diet are more than just trendy – they are downright powerful (9, 14). This diet, rich in colorful produce, olive oil, and lean proteins, fuels the body with essential nutrients while keeping harmful inflammation at bay. Here is a breakdown of the juicy evidence.

Nutritional Interventions: Food as Medicine

Imagine this: researchers dived into a smorgasbord of studies and found that good nutrition, especially through high-quality diets, can do wonders for your body (15). The results were not always carbon copies, but the trend was clear: better food equals stronger muscles, quicker steps, and an overall frailty downgrade. It is like upgrading your body's software – no bugs, just benefits!

Protein Power: Building Blocks of Strength

Protein is not just for bodybuilders. Turns out, it is also your best friend as you age. Studies show that eating more protein keeps frailty at bay by helping you maintain muscle mass and strength (16). So, whether it is a juicy steak, a hearty bowl of lentils, or a creamy yogurt, protein is like a gym membership for your muscles – without the sweaty fees.

Diet Quality: The VIP List of Foods

Not all diets are created equal. The higher the quality of your diet, the lower your chances of frailty. It is a simple formula: load up on fruits, veggies, whole grains, and healthy fats (hello, olive oil and avocado!), and your body will thank you. The Mediterranean diet is not just a buzzword; it is a ticket to feeling fabulous.

Antioxidants: Your Body's Defense Squad

Think of antioxidants as tiny warriors fighting off the damage that slows you down. A diet rich in antioxidants – like berries, spinach, and nuts – can help fend off frailty by tackling oxidative stress, which is just a fancy way of saying "body wear and tear." It is like giving your cells a spa day.

Long-Term Wins: Slow and Steady Pays Off

Good things come to those who stick with it. Long-term studies show that eating a high-quality diet over the years can delay frailty and keep your body and mind sharp. It is not just about a quick fix – it is about building a foundation for the future.

The Bottom Line: Eat Smart, Live Strong

At the end of the day, the recipe for avoiding frailty is deliciously simple. Add a generous serving of Mediterranean-style meals to your routine – think colorful fruits, crisp veggies, lean proteins, hearty whole grains, and luscious healthy fats. It is not just about surviving longer; it is about living better. So, grab that fork and dig into a healthier, happier you!

The Hidden Dangers of Ultra-Processed Foods

On the other hand, ultra-processed foods are like a double-edged sword—they offer convenience but come with significant downsides. These foods, which often include items like sugary snacks, instant noodles, and fast food, are designed to be quick and easy to consume. However, beneath this convenience lies a host of nutritional shortcomings.

These highly processed options are typically stripped of essential nutrients and packed with empty calories. It is like having a rusty shield that is incapable of providing real protection in the face of challenges. Instead of nourishing the body, ultra-processed foods are energy-dense, meaning they contain a lot of calories but very little in the way of vitamins, minerals, and other vital nutrients. When consumed regularly, these foods can wreak havoc on your health. They disrupt your body's metabolic processes, making it harder to maintain a healthy weight and manage blood sugar levels. Over time, this can lead to conditions such as obesity, diabetes mellitus, and heart disease (17). Additionally, the lack of proper nutrition weakens your body's natural defences, leaving you more vulnerable to illnesses and less capable of recovery and might cause frailty (18).

It is not just about the immediate effects, either. Consistently consuming ultra-processed foods can lead to long-term health issues. Your body's resilience—its ability to bounce back from stress and adversity—depends heavily on the quality of the fuel you provide it. Just as a car runs poorly on low-quality fuel, your body struggles to function optimally without the proper nutrients.

In essence, while ultra-processed foods might save time in the short term, they exact a heavy toll on your health in the long run. Making more mindful food choices can help you build a stronger, more resilient body capable of facing life's challenges with vigor and vitality.

The Microbiome Symphony

Deep within your gut resides a bustling city of microbes—the gut microbiome. It is no exaggeration to call it the unsung hero of health. This microbial metropolis thrives on dietary fiber from fruits and vegetables, producing beneficial compounds that influence everything from immune responses to mood regulation. A well-fed microbiome promotes resilience, while poor dietary choices—like low fiber intake—wreak havoc, exacerbating frailty (19).

Consider a study where older adults adopted a Mediterranean diet for a year. Their gut microbiomes shifted positively, reducing inflammation, and improving frailty markers (13). It is as if the orchestra gained a few virtuoso players, enhancing the entire performance.

Energy, Strength, and the Protein Connection

Protein is the star soloist in this symphony, crucial for maintaining muscle mass and strength. Unfortunately, many older adults consume insufficient protein, leading to muscle loss—a cornerstone of frailty. Increasing protein intake, particularly through lean meats, dairy, legumes, and nuts, has been shown to support muscle synthesis and counteract frailty

Vitamin D: The Sunshine Conductor

Vitamin D, synthesized from sunlight and fortified foods, acts like the lighting technician for the orchestra, ensuring every part is illuminated and functional. Low vitamin D levels are linked to higher frailty risk (20). While supplementation shows promise, it is crucial to pair it with a balanced diet for maximum benefit.

Personalized Nutrition

What if the secret to staying spry lies in a diet tailor-made just for you? Emerging research says we are onto something big: personalized dietary interventions could be the ultimate game-changer in the fight against frailty (9, 21). Tools like metabolomics and microbiome profiling enable tailored nutritional strategies (22), akin to handing the conductor a custom baton designed for each orchestra. Let us dig in (spoon first) to what the science says:

Custom-Made Menus: Because One Size Does not Fit All

Forget cookie-cutter diets – we are talking about crafting meal plans as unique as you are. Studies show that when older adults get diets tailored to their specific health needs, tastes, and routines, the results are positively delicious (23). Think better health outcomes with a side of satisfaction.

Supplements with a Personal Touch

Turns out, not all supplements are created equal. Personalized nutritional boosters designed to address your unique deficiencies can do wonders for muscle strength and physical function. Whether it is extra vitamin D, a protein boost, or something more exotic, these targeted tweaks pack a punch.

Lessons in Healthy Eating: A Recipe for Success

Imagine having a culinary coach teach you the ropes of balanced eating. Personalized dietary education helps older adults make smarter food choices, boosting their nutritional know-how and slashing frailty risk.

Playing the Long Game: Consistency is King

Stick with a personalized diet plan, and the benefits keep piling up. Long-term studies reveal that these custom interventions can stave off frailty and make life more enjoyable (13). Who would not want to age with grace (and good food)?

The Power Combo: Food, Fitness, and Friends

Why stop at personalized diets when you can pair them with exercise and a dash of social connection? This all-in-one approach has shown to be especially effective in tackling frailty. After all, life is better when you mix good food with good vibes.

The Takeaway: Personalized Nutrition for the Win

When it comes to preventing frailty, personalized dietary interventions are like bespoke suits for your health – they fit just right. By focusing on what makes each of us unique, these interventions promise to keep older adults healthier, happier, and more independent for longer. And honestly, who would not want a meal plan as special as they are?

2.2 Nutrition As A Modifiable Risk Factor

One of the most remarkable things about nutrition is its flexibility. While we cannot reverse the ticking clock or rewrite our genetic code, we hold the power to adjust what lands on our plates. This seemingly simple act can profoundly influence our health and vitality, especially as we age. Nutrition is not just about filling our stomachs—it is about fuelling our bodies with the premium ingredients they need to thrive.

The Mediterranean Diet: A Recipe for Resilience

Picture this: a dinner table adorned with vibrant salads, golden olive oil, flaky fish, hearty legumes, and crunchy nuts. This is not just a feast for the senses—it is a blueprint for better health. The Mediterranean diet, renowned for its heart-friendly and anti-inflammatory properties, has emerged as a nutritional champion in the fight against frailty.

What makes this diet so special? It is a synergy of nutrient-dense foods that work together to fortify your body. Olive oil, rich in monounsaturated fats, supports cardiovascular health. Fish provides omega-3 fatty acids that reduce inflammation and support brain function (23-25). Legumes and nuts deliver a powerful punch of protein and fiber, keeping muscles strong and digestion smooth.

But here is the kicker: adopting a Mediterranean-style diet is not about deprivation or strict rules. It is about abundance and enjoyment. Imagine swapping out that greasy fast food for a plate of grilled salmon with a side of roasted vegetables. Not only does your body get a premium fuel upgrade, but your taste buds thank you, too. Studies consistently show that adherence to this dietary pattern significantly lowers the risk of frailty (14). So, consider this your permission to savor life—one delicious bite at a time.

Protein: The Unsung Hero

Let us talk about protein—the unsung hero of nutrition. Think of protein as the scaffolding for your muscles. As we get older, our body's internal framework, or 'scaffolding,' starts to weaken due to a phenomenon known as 'anabolic resistance'. This term might sound complicated, but it essentially means that our muscles become less effective at utilizing protein to repair and grow. In simpler terms, even though we might be eating enough protein, our muscles are not as good at using it to stay strong and healthy. This decline in efficiency can lead to weaker muscles and decreased muscle mass over time. Here are a few key points and studies that highlight this phenomenon:

Age-Related Decline in Muscle Protein Synthesis: Research has shown that older adults experience a reduced rate of muscle protein synthesis in response to protein intake compared to younger individuals. This reduced ability to build and repair muscle is a hallmark of anabolic resistance (26).

Impact on Muscle Mass and Function: Anabolic resistance contributes to sarcopenia, which is the age-related loss of muscle mass and strength. This condition can lead to decreased mobility and increased risk of falls and fractures in older adults (27).

Mechanisms of Anabolic Resistance: Several factors contribute to anabolic resistance, including changes in muscle signaling pathways, reduced blood flow to muscles, and alterations in the digestive system that affect protein absorption (27).

Nutritional Interventions: Studies suggest that consuming higher-quality protein sources, increasing protein intake, and incorporating resistance exercise can help mitigate the effects of anabolic resistance in older adults (28).

So, maintaining muscle strength becomes more challenging as we age, but by understanding and addressing this phenomenon, we can better support muscle maintenance and overall health in older adults.

Here is the tricky part: older adults often do not consume enough protein. Whether it is due to changing appetites, dietary restrictions, or simply not knowing how much they need, the result is the same: muscle loss, weakness, and an increased risk of frailty. But the solution is within reach—and it is delicious.

Aim to include high-quality protein sources in every meal. Think eggs for breakfast, a hearty lentil soup for lunch, and a grilled chicken or tofu stir-fry for dinner. And do not forget snacks! A handful of almonds or a dollop of Greek yogurt can work wonders. The general guideline for older adults is around 1.2 to 1.5 grams of protein per kilogram of body weight daily. If math is not your thing, just remember this: prioritize protein, and your muscles will thank you.

Vitamin D: A Ray of Hope

Vitamin D is also known as the sunshine vitamin. It is not just about keeping your mood sunny; it is about fortifying your muscles and bones. Vitamin D plays a critical role in calcium absorption, which is essential for bone health. Without it, bones can become brittle, and the risk of fractures skyrockets—a serious concern for older adults.

Muscles love vitamin D, too. This vitamin helps them contract efficiently, improving balance and reducing the risk of falls. Unfortunately, many people, especially older adults, do not get enough vitamin D. Whether it is due to limited sun exposure, a diet lacking in fortified foods, or age-related declines in the skin's ability to produce vitamin D, the deficiency is common.

So, what is the fix? Spend some time in the sun—safely, of course—and consider incorporating vitamin D-rich foods like fatty fish, egg yolks, and fortified dairy into your diet. In some cases, supplements might be necessary, but always consult a healthcare provider first. Think of vitamin D as your body's secret weapon against frailty—a simple yet powerful ally in maintaining strength and resilience.

Antioxidants: Your Cellular Shield

Every day, our bodies wage a silent battle against oxidative stress, a process where unstable molecules called free radicals wreak havoc on cells. Over time, this damage accumulates and contributes to aging and frailty (29). But do not worry—you have got an army of antioxidants ready to fight back.

Antioxidants are like cellular superheroes, neutralizing free radicals and protecting your body from harm. You can find them in colorful fruits and vegetables, like berries, spinach, carrots, and bell peppers. These foods are not just a feast for the eyes; they are a defense system for your body. Take blueberries, for example. These tiny powerhouses are packed with anthocyanins, a type of antioxidant that supports brain and muscle health. Or consider spinach, loaded with vitamin C and beta-carotene, which help repair cellular damage. By eating a rainbow of fruits and vegetables, you are giving your body the tools it needs to stay strong and vibrant.

Practical Tips for Everyday Nutrition

Now that we have covered the science, let us talk practicality. Incorporating these nutritional principles into your daily life does not have to be complicated. Here are some simple tips to get you started:

Plan Your Meals: Take a few minutes each week to plan balanced meals. This not only ensures you are meeting your nutritional needs but also saves time and reduces stress.

Snack Smart: Keep healthy snacks on hand, like mixed nuts, fresh fruit, or whole-grain crackers with hummus. These are convenient and packed with nutrients.

Cook in Batches: Prepare larger portions of healthy dishes and store leftovers for easy meals throughout the week. Think soups, stews, and casseroles.

Experiment with Recipes: Try new recipes that feature Mediterranean ingredients or protein-rich foods. Cooking can be a fun and creative way to improve your diet.

Stay Hydrated: Do not forget to drink plenty of water. Proper hydration supports digestion, circulation, and overall well-being.

By making these small, intentional changes, you are not just modifying your diet—you are investing in your future. Nutrition truly is a modifiable risk factor, and with a little effort, you can harness its power to combat frailty and embrace a healthier, more resilient you.

2.3 Nutritional Strategies To Prevent Frailty

Prevention is better than cure, and when it comes to frailty, this adage could not be more true. A robust body and mind demand care, nourishment, and a dash of culinary creativity. Let us dive into some practical, science-backed nutritional strategies that are easy to adopt and crucial for warding off frailty. Here is your recipe for resilience:

Embrace Diversity: A Rainbow on Your Plate

A colorful plate is not just Instagram-worthy; it is a nutritional jackpot. Each hue in fruits and vegetables represents a unique set of nutrients working together to boost your health. Think of your meal as an artist's palette—the more colors, the richer the masterpiece (your health, in this case!).

The Power of Colors

Red (tomatoes, strawberries): Packed with lycopene and anthocyanins, these fight inflammation and protect your heart.

Orange and Yellow (carrots, bell peppers): Rich in beta-carotene and vitamin C, which promote immune health and skin resilience.

Green (spinach, broccoli): Loaded with folate, iron, and antioxidants to strengthen bones and muscles.

Blue and Purple (blueberries, eggplant): These hues bring anthocyanins that support brain health and combat oxidative stress.

White and Brown (onions, mushrooms): Often underrated, these contribute fiber, selenium, and phytonutrients.

Tips to Embrace Diversity

- Swap the boring side salad for a vibrant medley of roasted veggies.

- Experiment with lesser-known fruits like dragon fruit or persimmon.

- Keep frozen mixed vegetables on hand for quick stir-fries or soups.

- Remember, variety is not just the spice of life—it is the foundation of good health.

Prioritize Protein: The Building Block Bonanza

Protein is not just for bodybuilders. For older adults, it is the secret to maintaining strength and vitality. Think of protein as the scaffolding holding your body together. Without it, muscles weaken, and frailty creeps in.

Protein Powerhouses

Animal Sources: Lean meats, fish, eggs, and dairy are rich in complete proteins, providing all essential amino acids.

Plant Sources: Legumes, tofu, quinoa, and nuts cater to those aiming for a more plant-based diet.

Pro Tips for Protein

Pair It with Resistance Training: Imagine protein as bricks and exercise as the mortar. Together, they build a sturdy structure—your muscles.

Space It Out: Instead of a protein bomb at dinner, aim to distribute intake evenly across meals.

Snack Smarter: Swap chips for a handful of almonds or a hard-boiled egg.

Supplements to the Rescue: For those struggling to meet their protein needs, especially frail individuals, supplements can fill the gap. Consult a healthcare provider for options tailored to you.

Limit Ultra-Processed Foods: Break Up with Junk

If ultra-processed foods were a person, they would be that incredibly charming yet undeniably toxic partner everyone warns you about. They sweep you off your feet with their convenience and tantalizing flavors, making life seem easier and more enjoyable. Like a partner who always knows just what to say to make you smile, these foods are designed to be irresistible, drawing you in with their bright packaging and instant gratification. However, beneath that appealing exterior lies a different story. Just like a toxic relationship can chip away at your well-being over time, ultra-processed foods wreak havoc on your health. While they might seem like a quick solution to hunger, they are essentially empty promises —devoid of the essential nutrients your body needs to thrive. Instead, they are packed with unhealthy fats, sugars, and additives that can lead to serious health issues. Regularly consuming these foods is akin to being in a relationship that drains your energy and leaves you feeling worse over time. They disrupt your metabolic processes, contribute to weight gain, and increase the risk of chronic diseases such as diabetes mellitus, heart disease, and even certain cancers. Your body, much like your emotional health in a toxic relationship, becomes less resilient and more susceptible to harm.

In the end, while ultra-processed foods might offer temporary pleasure, their long-term impact on your health is anything but pleasant. It is vital to recognize their true nature and make mindful choices that prioritize your well-being. Just as you would eventually walk away from a toxic partner for the sake of your happiness and health, it is wise to distance yourself from these foods and embrace a diet rich in whole, nourishing foods. Your body will thank you for it, rewarding you with better health and greater vitality.

The Hidden Dangers

- Packed with sugar, salt, and unhealthy fats, they are calorie-dense but nutrient-poor.

- Regular consumption contributes to inflammation, weight gain, and even cognitive decline —all precursors to frailty.

Simple Swaps to Shine

Snacks: Choose fresh fruit, nuts, or Greek yogurt over candy bars and chips.

Meals: Opt for homemade soups, stews, or salads instead of pre-packaged meals.

Drinks: Replace sugary sodas with sparkling water infused with citrus or berries.

Cooking at home does not need to be a chore. Batch cook soups or stews, freeze portions, and embrace the simplicity of one-pot meals. Even a little effort can go a long way in cutting down on ultra-processed food intake.

Hydration Matters: Do not Dry Out

Dehydration often sneaks up on older adults, leading to fatigue, confusion, and even falls. Staying hydrated is one of the simplest ways to maintain vitality and fend off frailty.

Signs of Dehydration

- Dry mouth or lips

- Dizziness or light-headedness

- Dark urine or infrequent urination

Hydration Hacks

Sip Throughout the Day: Keep a water bottle within reach and take small sips regularly.

Make It Tasty: Add a splash of fruit juice, a wedge of lemon, or a few mint leaves to your water.

Eat Your Water: Water-rich foods like cucumbers, melons, and oranges add hydration and nutrients.

Avoid Overhydration

While rare, overhydration can dilute essential minerals in your body. Drink according to thirst and activity levels. Hydration is not just about water. Soups, herbal teas, and even fruits and vegetables play a role in keeping your cells plump and happy.

These strategies, while simple, can make a profound difference when tailored to individual needs. Older adults often face challenges like reduced appetite, dental issues, or limited mobility. By understanding their unique circumstances, caregivers and loved ones can turn these nutritional principles into achievable, everyday habits. After all, the goal is not just to live longer—it is to live better.

2.4 Chronic Conditions, Frailty, And Nutrition

Frailty rarely travels alone. Like an uninvited guest at a party, it brings along its close companions: chronic conditions such as diabetes mellitus, cardiovascular disease, and obesity. Together, they create a troublesome trio that wreaks havoc on the health and well-being of older adults. But here is the silver lining: nutrition is not just a supporting actor in this story – it is the hero that can turn the tide. Let us dive into how the right food choices can disrupt this vicious cycle, one meal at a time.

Diabetes mellitus: Keeping Blood Sugar in Check

Think of diabetes mellitus (DM) and frailty as two rivals egging each other on. When blood sugar levels spiral out of control, complications like nerve damage, poor circulation, and muscle weakness pave the way for frailty. On the flip side, frailty's physical and metabolic changes make managing diabetes even trickier.

The solution? A balanced diet that plays referee. Swap refined carbs (yes, those tempting cookies and pastries) for whole grains like oats and quinoa. Load up on colorful vegetables – they are not just pretty to look at but also rich in fiber, which helps stabilize blood sugar levels. And do not forget protein; lean options like chicken, fish, and legumes keep muscles strong and your energy steady.

A dash of spice can also do wonders. Cinnamon, for instance, may help improve insulin sensitivity (30), while turmeric's active ingredient, curcumin, fights inflammation (31). Of course, moderation is key – a sprinkle, not a flood!

In essence, managing diabetes mellitus through nutrition is not about deprivation; it is about making smarter, tastier choices. It is a delicious way to keep frailty at bay while enjoying your meals guilt-free.

Cardiovascular Disease: Heart-Healthy Choices

Your heart works tirelessly, but frailty and cardiovascular disease (CVD) can make its job feel like running a marathon uphill. Poor diet choices – think salty chips and greasy burgers – act like speed bumps, slowing down recovery and resilience.

Enter the Mediterranean diet, a culinary love letter to your heart. With its generous servings of olive oil, nuts, seeds, and fatty fish, this diet is packed with omega-3 fatty acids that reduce inflammation and improve heart health. Swap your butter for avocado slices, your soda for a glass of water infused with lemon, and watch your heart say, "Thank you!" Fruits and vegetables, particularly leafy greens, and berries, are your heart's best friends. Rich in antioxidants, they act like a cleanup crew, mopping up harmful free radicals. And do not underestimate the power of garlic – its natural compounds can help lower blood pressure and cholesterol levels.

Even chocolate makes an appearance in this heart-health journey. Dark chocolate (the real deal, not the sugary imposters) contains flavonoids that improve blood flow. A square or two after dinner? Yes, please.

Obesity: A Balancing Act

Obesity and frailty may seem like polar opposites, but they are often two sides of the same coin. Excess weight strains joints, saps energy, and fuels inflammation, while frailty exacerbates mobility issues and muscle loss. It is a complicated dance, but the right nutrition can help you lead.

Contrary to popular belief, tackling obesity is not just about eating less – it is about eating better. Nutrient-dense foods, such as salmon, spinach, and almonds, provide essential vitamins and minerals without empty calories. Aim for meals that focus on building muscle, not just burning fat. Think grilled chicken salads with a sprinkle of seeds, or quinoa bowls loaded with roasted veggies and a dollop of hummus.

Hydration also plays a starring role. Often, we mistake thirst for hunger, leading to unnecessary snacking. A glass of water before meals can curb overeating and keep you feeling refreshed.

And let us not forget portion control – the art of savouring rather than scarfing. Using smaller plates, eating mindfully, and tuning into hunger cues can make a world of difference. It is not about dieting; it is about redefining your relationship with food.

The Gut Microbiome: Your Tiny Allies

Beneath the surface lies a bustling community of microorganisms – your gut microbiome. These tiny allies have a big role in your health, influencing everything from digestion to inflammation and even frailty.

The key to a happy gut? Prebiotics and probiotics. Prebiotics, found in foods like bananas, onions, and asparagus, feed the good bacteria in your gut. Probiotics, on the other hand, introduce beneficial bacteria. Think yogurt, kefir, sauerkraut, and miso soup.

Diversity is essential. Imagine your gut as a vibrant garden, the more variety in your diet, the more diverse and resilient your microbiome. Fermented foods, whole grains, and fiber-rich fruits and veggies create the perfect ecosystem. Research also points to the potential of gut-brain communication. A healthy microbiome might not only reduce frailty (19) but also boost mood and cognitive function. It is a win-win for body and mind (32, 33).

In brief, nutrition is the ultimate game-changer in the battle against frailty and chronic conditions. It is the sword that cuts through complications and the shield that fortifies resilience. By making thoughtful, tasty choices – whether it is adding a handful of nuts to your salad, swapping soda for green tea, or experimenting with a new spice – you are not just eating for survival; you are eating for strength, vitality, and joy. Frailty and chronic conditions may crash the party, but with nutrition as your ally, you are the life of the feast. So, grab your fork, dig in, and savor the journey to a healthier, happier you.

CHAPTER 3: MACRONUTRIENTS AND FRAILTY

What you eat can play a protector role in building resilience against frailty. Imagine your plate as a battlefield, where macronutrients—protein, carbohydrates, and fats—are your trusty allies, ready to fight for your health and vitality. In this chapter, we will unravel the fascinating ways these nutrients impact frailty prevention and management, ensuring you are not just surviving but thriving. Let us dive into their roles and learn how to power up our golden years with every bite.

3.1 Role Of Protein In Frailty

If macronutrients were Marvel characters, protein would undoubtedly be Captain America. Why? Because it is the ultimate builder and protector of muscle—a key player in preventing frailty (34). But unlike the fictional superhero, protein does not just swoop in for dramatic battles; it is there for the quiet, everyday victories, showing up at breakfast, lunch, and dinner to keep you strong and steady.

The Muscle Maker

Proteins are the body's construction crew, made up of amino acids that rebuild muscles after the wear and tear of daily life. Picture them with hard hats and tool belts, patching up the micro-tears in your muscles after a walk, a workout, or even just carrying groceries. As we age, however, our body's workforce becomes a little less efficient. This slowdown, known as anabolic resistance, means that older adults need more protein to achieve the same muscle-strengthening effects as their younger selves.

Protein's Frailty-Fighting Arsenal

So, what makes protein such a game-changer in the fight against frailty? For starters, it helps preserve muscle mass and strength, two critical factors for maintaining mobility and independence. Without enough protein, the body starts to cannibalize its own muscle tissue, leading to weakness and a greater risk of falls and injuries.

But not all proteins are created equal. While animal proteins like chicken, fish, and dairy are rich in essential amino acids, they can sometimes come with a catch. Diets high in animal protein have been linked to increased dietary acid load, which may negatively impact overall health in some older adults. On the flip side, plant-based proteins from sources like lentils, beans, and nuts offer muscle-building benefits without the acid load, along with added perks like fiber and antioxidants. Think of plant-based proteins as the eco-friendly option—powerful yet gentle on the system.

How Much Protein is Enough?

Here is where the numbers come in handy. Experts suggest older adults aim for 1.0-1.2 grams of protein per kilogram of body weight daily. For a 70-kg person, that is about 70-84 grams of protein—the equivalent of three eggs at breakfast, a chicken breast at lunch, and a hearty lentil soup at dinner.

Timing is just as important as quantity. Instead of loading up on protein at one meal, spread it evenly throughout the day to maximize muscle protein synthesis. Imagine your muscles as a sponge—they can only soak up so much protein at once, so regular "watering" is key.

Practical Tips for Protein Power

Getting enough protein does not have to be a chore. Here are some easy and delicious ways to boost your intake:

Start Strong: Kick off your day with a protein-packed breakfast. Think scrambled eggs with spinach, Greek yogurt with a sprinkle of nuts, or a protein smoothie with your favorite fruits.

Snack Smart: Swap out chips and cookies for protein-rich snacks like cheese sticks, roasted chickpeas, or a handful of almonds.

Go Global: Explore cuisines that celebrate protein. Indian dals, Mediterranean hummus, and Japanese edamame are flavourful ways to diversify your sources.

Mix It Up: Combine animal and plant proteins in your meals. A chicken salad with quinoa or a beef stir-fry with tofu not only boosts your intake but also adds variety.

Beyond Muscles: Protein's Hidden Talents

While protein's role in muscle health gets the spotlight, its benefits do not stop there. Protein also supports immune function, aids in wound healing, and even helps regulate hormones. It is the unsung hero working behind the scenes to keep your body running smoothly.

In the battle against frailty, protein is your steadfast ally—ready to rebuild, repair, and reinforce. So, go ahead and embrace this mighty macronutrient. Your muscles, bones, and future self will thank you for it.

3.2 Carbohydrates And Energy Balance

Carbohydrates often get a bad rap, but let us set the record straight: they are not the villain of this story. In fact, carbs are more like the reliable sidekick—steadily providing energy to keep you moving, thinking, and thriving. In the quest to combat frailty, carbohydrates are an unsung hero that deserves a standing ovation.

The Energy Equation

Carbohydrates are your body's go-to energy source. They are broken down into glucose, a type of sugar that fuels your cells, muscles, and brain. Imagine glucose as the premium gas that powers your body's engine. For older adults, maintaining this energy balance is especially crucial. Why? Because frailty often sneaks in alongside unintentional weight loss, fatigue, and reduced physical activity.

Quality Over Quantity: Not All Carbs Are Created Equal

Here is where it gets interesting. While all carbs provide energy, their quality can vary drastically. Think of carbs as a spectrum: on one end, you have complex carbohydrates like whole grains, fruits, and vegetables—nutrient-packed powerhouses rich in fiber. On the other end, you have got refined carbs like sugary cereals and white bread—quick fixes that lead to energy spikes followed by inevitable crashes.

Complex carbs are the golden trio for older adults. Fiber, a standout nutrient in these carbs, not only supports digestion but also stabilizes blood sugar levels and reduces inflammation —a key factor in frailty (35). Meanwhile, refined carbs can act like party crashers, contributing to inflammation and leaving you feeling drained. It is a no-brainer: choose the good guys.

Carbs, Fibers and Frailty: The Research Rundown

What does science say? While there is no direct link between total carbohydrate intake and frailty over time, studies highlight the importance of carb quality (36). Eating a diet high in fiber has been consistently linked to a lower risk of becoming frail. A study found that older adults who consumed a lot of fiber had a lower chance of frailty compared to those who ate less fiber (37). This suggests that getting enough fiber might be a good way to help prevent frailty in older adults. Additionally, a thorough review of multiple clinical trials indicated that good nutrition, including eating more fiber, can help manage and reduce frailty (9). This review emphasized the importance of proper nutrition for keeping the body strong and functioning well. These findings highlight the importance of including fiber-rich foods in our diets. Regularly eating these foods can lead to better physical health and resilience as we get older. It also means that it is not just about eating carbohydrates; it is about choosing the right kinds of carbs.

Fiber is essential for maintaining good digestion and regular bowel movements, which can be particularly important as we age. It helps to prevent constipation, which can be a common issue for older adults. Fiber also helps to regulate blood sugar levels, which can be beneficial for those at risk of or managing diabetes mellitus. Additionally, a diet high in fiber can help to lower cholesterol levels, reducing the risk of heart disease. Foods like fruits, vegetables, whole grains, and legumes are not only delicious but also help support overall health and strength in older adults. By including more fiber-rich foods in your diet, you are not only helping to prevent frailty but also supporting overall health. Fiber helps to keep you feeling full and satisfied, which can aid in maintaining a healthy weight. This is important because carrying excess weight can put additional strain on your joints and muscles, leading to an increased risk of frailty and other health issues.

In brief, fiber plays a key role in maintaining good health and preventing frailty as we age. By choosing the right kinds of carbs, like those found in fruits, vegetables, whole grains, and legumes, you can support your body's overall strength and resilience. So, make sure to include plenty of fiber-rich foods in your diet to stay healthy and strong.

Finding Your Carb Sweet Spot

So, how much carbohydrate is the right amount? Experts recommend that carbs make up about 45-65% of your daily caloric intake. For someone consuming 2000 calories a day, this translates to 225-325 grams of carbohydrates. But remember, it is the quality that counts. A bowl of steel-cut oats topped with fresh berries is a far better choice than a doughnut dunked in sugary glaze.

Practical Tips for Carb Success

Upgrade Your Breakfast: Swap out sugary cereals for oatmeal or whole-grain toast with avocado.

Sneak in Veggies: Add spinach or kale to your pasta sauce and grated carrots to your casseroles.

Snack Wisely: Munch on sliced apples with peanut butter or whole-grain crackers with hummus.

Experiment with Grains: Try quinoa, farro, or bulgur for a change from rice and pasta. Quinoa, farro, and bulgur are all nutritious and versatile grains, each offering unique benefits. Quinoa is a complete protein and gluten-free, making it an exceptional choice for those seeking a quick-cooking, nutrient-dense option with a mild, nutty flavor. Farro is rich in fiber, protein, and essential nutrients, known for its chewy texture and nutty taste, but takes longer to cook and is not gluten-free. Bulgur, with its mild flavor and soft texture, cooks quickly and is a great addition to Middle Eastern dishes. Each grain supports overall health and can be a valuable part of a balanced diet, whether you are looking for convenience, heartiness, or specific dietary needs.

Beyond Energy: Carbs as Brain Boosters

Here is a fun fact: your brain runs almost exclusively on glucose, which is a type of sugar that comes from the carbs you eat. So, the carbs you consume directly affect how well your brain works. This is especially important for older adults.

Studies have shown that eating nutrient-rich carbs, like those found in fruits, vegetables, and whole grains, can help keep your brain sharp (38). These healthy carbs provide a steady supply of glucose, which your brain needs to function properly. On the other hand, eating too many refined carbs, like sugary snacks and white bread, can lead to spikes and crashes in blood sugar levels, which can negatively impact your cognitive function. For older adults, choosing the right kind of carbs can support mental sharpness, memory, and overall brain health. Research suggests that a diet rich in whole, nutrient-dense carbs can help improve memory and reduce the risk of cognitive decline . One study found that older adults who followed a Mediterranean diet, which is high in healthy carbs, had better cognitive function and a lower risk of developing Alzheimer's disease (25).

Briefly, the carbs you eat play a key role in brain health and they are the quiet yet essential players in the fight against frailty. They provide the energy to fuel your days and the nutrients to support long-term health. So, the next time someone tells you to cut out carbs, remind them that your body and brain need these vital nutrients—and you are making the smart, healthy choices to get the best out of them.

3.3 Fats And Their Effect

Fat: the misunderstood macronutrient. For years, it has been accused of crimes against health—clogging arteries, expanding waistlines, and generally being a dietary villain. But the truth? Fat is not the foe; it is the firefighter, dousing the flames of inflammation and helping you maintain overall health. Like any firefighter, though, the type of fat you call upon makes all the difference.

Good Fats vs. Bad Fats

Let us get one thing straight: not all fats are created equal. Imagine fats as characters in a story—unsaturated fats are the heroes, always ready to swoop in and save the day. Found in avocados, nuts, seeds, and olive oil, these fats are anti-inflammatory and heart-healthy, working tirelessly to protect your brain and body from the ravages of aging.

On the other hand, saturated and trans fats are the villains of this tale. Lurking in processed foods, fried snacks, and fatty cuts of meat, they stoke the fires of inflammation and increase the risk of chronic diseases like diabetes, heart disease, and cognitive decline. Think of them as the troublemakers who leave chaos in their wake, undoing all the good work your body's trying to accomplish.

So, what is the secret to navigating this complex cast of characters? It is simple: choose your fats wisely. Make room for the heroes on your plate and leave the villains out of your pantry.

The Role of Fat in Frailty

Here is where it gets interesting. While the total amount of fat you eat does not seem to have a direct link to frailty, the type of fat you consume plays a critical role. Research has shown that monounsaturated fats—the kind found in olive oil and avocados—are particularly beneficial (39, 40). They help maintain physical health, cognitive function, and even reduce the risk of inflammation—a key factor in frailty.

But fats can be a double-edged sword. Excessive consumption of animal-based fats, like those in fatty cuts of meat and butter, may increase frailty scores over time. This does not mean you have to swear off your favorite steak dinner, but moderation is key. Balancing your fat intake with plenty of fruits, vegetables, and whole grains can tip the scales in your favor.

The Goldilocks Zone

So, how much fat is just right? Experts recommend that fats make up 20-35% of your daily caloric intake. For someone eating 2000 calories a day, that is about 44-78 grams. But remember, not all grams are equal—quality matters more than quantity. Picture this: you are building a house. Would you rather use sturdy bricks or flimsy cardboard? The same logic applies to fats. Sturdy, high-quality fats from whole food sources like nuts, seeds, and fatty fish provide lasting benefits, while processed and fried foods offer little more than a quick fix and long-term harm.

Practical Tips for Fabulous Fats

Incorporating healthy fats into your diet does not have to be complicated. Here are some easy and delicious ways to up your fat game:

Avocado Awesomeness: Add avocado slices to your sandwiches, mash them into guacamole, or blend them into smoothies for a creamy, nutrient-packed treat.

Nutty Delights: Snack on a handful of almonds or walnuts. They are not just tasty; they are loaded with omega-3s and antioxidants.

Oil Upgrade: Swap vegetable oil for olive oil in your cooking and salad dressings. It is a simple switch with big health payoffs.

Go Fish: Incorporate fatty fishlike salmon, mackerel, or sardines into your meals twice a week. These seafood stars are rich in omega-3 fatty acids, which are anti-inflammatory and brain-boosting.

Ditch the Processed Stuff: Say goodbye to chips and cookies. Instead, reach for whole foods that satisfy your cravings and nourish your body.

Beyond Frailty: The Bigger Picture

Healthy fats are not just about fighting frailty; they are about supporting every system in your body. From aiding in hormone production to ensuring your skin stays radiant, fats are the multitaskers of the nutrition world. They help your body absorb fat-soluble vitamins like A, D, E, and K, making sure you get the most out of every bite you take.

By choosing the right fats, you are not just feeding your body; you are fuelling a future of resilience and vitality. So, drizzle that olive oil, scoop that avocado, and savor that salmon—your body will thank you, today and every day.

3.4 Optimal Macronutrients For Frail Adults

If macronutrients were a band, balance would be their chart-topping hit. Each macronutrient—protein, carbohydrates, and fats—has a unique role to play, but getting the mix just right is the secret to optimizing nutrition for frail individuals. Think of it as crafting the perfect harmony: every note counts, and together, they create something powerful.

Building the Plate

Let us break it down into manageable bites—literally. Your plate can become a tool for resilience when you focus on the right macronutrient distribution:

Protein Power: Protein should be the star of the show, contributing about 25-30% of your daily calories. Why? Because protein builds and repairs muscle, which is essential for maintaining mobility and independence. Lean meats, fish, eggs, legumes, and dairy products are excellent options. Do not forget plant-based sources like tofu, lentils, and quinoa—they pack a protein punch with added fiber benefits.

Carb Comfort: Carbs provide the energy you need to power through your day, making them the foundation of your plate at 45-55% of daily calories. Prioritize complex carbohydrates from whole grains, fruits, and vegetables. They release energy slowly, keeping your blood sugar steady and your body fuelled for longer.

Fantastic Fats: Healthy fats round out your plate, contributing 20-30% of daily calories. These fats, found in nuts, seeds, avocados, and fatty fish, are essential for brain health, hormone production, and reducing inflammation. Say yes to olive oil drizzles and almond butter spreads!

Timing Matters

It is not just what you eat but when you eat it. Frail adults often find large meals daunting, so distributing macronutrients across smaller, more frequent meals can help. Think of it as keeping a steady flow of fuel to your body's engine.

Start your day with a balanced breakfast—perhaps a bowl of oatmeal topped with nuts and berries. Follow it up with a mid-morning snack of yogurt or cheese. For lunch and dinner, aim for a protein, a complex carb, and a healthy fat, like grilled chicken with quinoa and a side of roasted veggies. Sprinkle in a few light snacks to keep hunger and fatigue at bay.

Tailoring to Needs

Here is the golden rule: nutrition is not one-size-fits-all. Your optimal macronutrient ratio depends on factors like your body weight, activity level, and any existing health conditions. For instance, someone recovering from illness may need more protein, while a person with diabetes might focus on controlling their carb intake. This is where a dietitian becomes your best ally. They can help design a plan that is as unique as you are, ensuring you get the right nutrients in the right amounts. Think of it as having a personal nutrition coach cheering you on.

CHAPTER 4: MICRONUTRIENTS AND FRAILTY

Frailty does not happen overnight. It creeps in over time, often without notice. What if the secret to slowing it down lies in the smallest things we often overlook? Enter micronutrients: the vitamins, minerals, and antioxidants that work quietly behind the scenes to keep us strong, sharp, and resilient. This chapter dives into the outsized role of these tiny nutrients in maintaining health and combating frailty. Let us unravel their mysteries one by one.

4.1 Vitamins And Their Role

Picture vitamins as the backstage crew of a theatre production. You might not see them in action, but without them, the whole show could fall apart. In the story of frailty, vitamins are the unsung heroes supporting your bones, brain, and immune defences. Let us spotlight some of the key players:

Bone Health: The Calcium-Enabler, Vitamin D

Vitamin D is the body's sunshine-powered superstar. It helps you absorb calcium, the mineral that keeps your bones sturdy enough to support your every move. A lack of vitamin D is like forgetting the glue in a craft project — things start falling apart, leading to brittle bones and fractures. Think of it as your bones' personal cheerleader, urging calcium to do its thing.

But here is the kicker: many older adults do not get enough vitamin D. Why? Aging skin produces less of it, and who really wants to sit in the sun for hours when a comfy chair and a book are calling? Plus, modern life often keeps us indoors. That is why a little supplement might just be your bones' best friend. Pair it with calcium-rich foods like dairy, leafy greens, or fortified plant-based milk for a bone-building tag team. Want an extra tip? A walk in the sun not only boosts vitamin D levels but can also lift your mood. Double win!

Cognitive Health: The Brain-Boosting B-Vitamins

Ever had a moment where you walk into a room and forget why you are there? While some forgetfulness is normal, deficiencies in B vitamins like B6, B12, and folate can make your memory foggy. These vitamins help your brain process information and stay sharp. They are like a power-up in a video game, giving your neurons the boost they need to keep firing.

For older adults, B12 deficiency is particularly sneaky. It often hides behind vague symptoms like fatigue, numbness, and memory issues. What is worse? The body's ability to absorb B12 from food declines with age. That is where fortified cereals, eggs, fish, or a daily supplement come in to save the day.

B6 and folate are equally crucial. They help produce neurotransmitters—the brain's messengers—and reduce levels of homocysteine, a compound linked to cognitive decline. To give your brain a helping hand, dig into foods like bananas, avocados, spinach, and beans. Remember: a well-fed brain is a happy brain.

Immune Health: The Infection Fighter, Vitamin C

Remember the age-old advice to drink orange juice when you are sick? That is thanks to vitamin C. This mighty nutrient keeps your immune system ready to tackle invaders, whether it is a common cold or a more serious infection. For frail adults, a strong immune system can mean the difference between bouncing back quickly or struggling for weeks.

Vitamin C works as a shield, neutralizing free radicals that can damage cells. It is also a key player in collagen production, which helps wounds heal faster. Think of it as your personal bodyguard, always on duty. Adding citrus fruits, bell peppers, strawberries, or even a vitamin C supplement to your diet is an easy way to bolster your defences. Pro tip: a colorful plate is not just pretty to look at; it is likely packed with this immune-boosting nutrient.

Tying It All Together

Vitamins may be tiny, but their impact on health is anything but. From keeping your bones strong and your mind sharp to defending your body against invaders, these micronutrients are your silent allies in the fight against frailty. So, the next time you are planning a meal or popping a supplement, remember: you are fuelling your body's backstage crew. And with them working tirelessly, the show of life goes on—vibrantly and resiliently.

4.2 Minerals And Their Influence On Frailty Markers

If vitamins are the backstage crew, minerals are the orchestra. Together, they create harmony in your body, keeping everything in sync. But when they are out of tune, frailty markers like muscle weakness, fatigue, and poor mobility start to show. Let us meet the standout minerals that hit all the right notes:

Calcium: The Bone Builder

Calcium is often touted as the go-to nutrient for bone health, but its influence extends beyond just keeping your skeleton strong. Think of it as the foundation of movement. Your muscles depend on calcium to contract and relax smoothly, much like a well-oiled hinge on a door. Without enough calcium, you might feel crampy, weak, or even unsteady — like a car sputtering to the finish line. Study suggests that having low bone mineral density (BMD) might increase the risk of frailty. However, we need more research to confirm this link (41).

Here is the twist: many older adults do not get enough calcium. Whether it is due to avoiding dairy or simply overlooking calcium-rich foods, the result is the same — weaker bones and reduced mobility.

But fear not! Calcium is not exclusive to milk and cheese. Leafy greens like kale and collard greens, crunchy almonds, and fortified plant-based milks can step in to save the day. So, whether you are sipping on almond milk or tossing spinach into your salad, you are giving your bones the building blocks they need.

Phosphorous: The Companion to Calcium

Phosphorous is an important mineral that our body needs for many different functions. It helps to form strong bones and teeth, and it is also necessary for making proteins that help grow, maintain, and repair cells and tissues. Phosphorous plays a key role in producing ATP (adenosine triphosphate), which is the molecule our body uses to store and use energy. It is also involved in important bodily functions like kidney function, muscle movements, a normal heartbeat, and sending signals through the nerves.

Phosphorus, alongside calcium, forms an effective and dynamic duo. Calcium provides the structural strength for bones, while phosphorous ensures that the bones are formed correctly and stay healthy. This duo is necessary for maintaining bone health throughout life, especially as we age, and our bones become more susceptible to weakening. You can find phosphorous in a variety of foods, including meat, poultry, fish, dairy products, eggs, nuts, legumes, and whole grains.

Magnesium: The Muscle Whisperer

If calcium is the builder, magnesium is the project manager, ensuring everything runs smoothly. This mineral is crucial for muscle function and relaxation. Imagine it as a soothing massage for your insides, preventing cramps, spasms, and that stiff, achy feeling after a long day. But magnesium does not stop there. It is also a key player in maintaining your energy levels and regulating sleep. And let us face it — a good night's sleep can do wonders for frailty prevention. Think of magnesium as a double-duty nutrient: it keeps your body active during the day and helps you recharge at night.

Where can you find this miracle mineral? Look no further than nuts, seeds, and whole grains. A handful of almonds or sunflower seeds could be your ticket to better muscle health and a restful night. And if you are feeling adventurous, try cooking with quinoa or sprinkling flaxseeds on your morning yogurt for an extra magnesium boost.

Iron: The Energy Driver

Feeling tired even after a full eight hours of sleep? You are not alone. Iron deficiency is a common cause behind unexplained fatigue, especially in older adults. Think of iron as the fuel your body needs to keep moving. It carries oxygen in your blood, delivering it to every cell in your body. Without enough iron, you are essentially running on empty, and that lack of energy can fast-track frailty.

The good news? Iron is easy to add to your diet. Red meat is a classic source, but plant-based options like lentils, beans, and spinach are just as effective. Here is a pro tip: pair iron-rich foods with vitamin C to enhance absorption. For instance, a spinach salad with a squeeze of lemon juice or a bowl of lentil soup with a side of orange slices can work wonders. It is like giving your body a one-two punch of nutrients to keep fatigue at bay.

Zinc: The Healer

Let us not forget zinc, the unsung hero of mineral health. This trace mineral plays a vital role in wound healing, immune support, and overall cellular function. Think of it as the repair crew that steps in when things go wrong. For frail individuals, quicker recovery times and a robust immune system are game-changers.

Oysters might be the richest source of zinc, but if seafood is not your thing, no worries! You can find zinc in lean meats, chickpeas, pumpkin seeds, and even dark chocolate. Yes, you read that right — a little square of dark chocolate can be both a treat and a health boost.

Potassium: The Balancer

Last but not least, potassium deserves a standing ovation. This mineral helps balance fluids and electrolytes in your body, keeping your blood pressure in check and reducing the risk of muscle cramps. Potassium is like the stage manager, ensuring everything behind the scenes runs seamlessly.

Bananas might be potassium's poster child, but do not overlook other sources like sweet potatoes, avocados, and beans. A baked sweet potato topped with avocado slices can be a potassium-packed meal that is as delicious as it is nutritious.

Bringing It All Together

Minerals might be small, but their impact on frailty markers is anything but minor. From building strong bones to fuelling your muscles and boosting energy, these nutrients play a pivotal role in keeping you active and resilient. So, the next time you are grocery shopping, think of your cart as a symphony, filled with the harmonious notes of calcium, magnesium, iron, zinc, and potassium. Your body will thank you for it. However, the impact of taking mineral supplements on muscle loss and frailty is still unclear (42). This means we need personalized nutrition plans. Future research should focus on well-structured clinical trials to better understand how minerals can improve muscle health and function. This will help provide clearer advice for healthcare practices.

4.3 Antioxidants And Their Role

Imagine your body as a bustling city. Oxidative stress is like the pollution that builds up from all the hustle and bustle—pesky free radicals running amok, causing chaos. Enter antioxidants, the heroic cleanup crew, swooping in to neutralize these harmful molecules and keep the city's operations running smoothly. Recent studies suggest that antioxidants can help prevent cell damage by stopping free radicals from spreading or forming. This can reduce oxidative stress, boost the immune system, and promote a longer, healthier life (43). Let us explore how these micronutrient superheroes work their magic and why they are essential for your health.

The Antioxidant Trio: Vitamins A, C, and E

Meet the Antioxidant Trio—Vitamins A, C, and E. These vitamins work together like a superhero team, fighting oxidative damage that can lead to frailty (44).

Vitamin A: The sharp-eyed archer of the group, Vitamin A, is crucial for maintaining healthy vision. It also supports your immune system and helps your organs function properly. You can find Vitamin A in foods like carrots, sweet potatoes, and leafy greens. So, munching on these colorful veggies is like giving your eyes a power boost and keeping frailty at bay!

Vitamin C: The defender with the invincible shield, Vitamin C, powers your immune system and accelerates wound healing. It is also a potent antioxidant that protects cells from oxidative stress. Citrus fruits like oranges, strawberries, and kiwi are rich in Vitamin C. Think of them as your body's daily dose of defense.

Vitamin E: The protector of cells, Vitamin E, prevents cellular damage caused by free radicals. It is particularly good at safeguarding your skin and other tissues. Nuts, seeds, and green leafy vegetables are great sources of Vitamin E. Incorporating these into your diet is like reinforcing your body's defences.

Together, these vitamins form a formidable team, warding off the oxidative damage that can lead to frailty. Think of antioxidant-rich foods like your body's built-in repair shop, keeping everything in top working order.

Polyphenols: Nature's Secret Weapon

Next up, we have polyphenols—nature's secret weapon. Polyphenols are a group of natural compounds found in plants, categorized into flavonoids, phenolic acids, stilbenes, and lignans. Collectively, these compounds are known as phytochemicals. They help neutralize harmful free radicals, reducing oxidative stress and potentially lowering the risk of chronic diseases like heart disease, diabetes mellitus, and certain cancers. Additionally, polyphenols can reduce inflammation in the body, which is linked to many chronic illnesses. They also promote the growth of beneficial gut bacteria, supporting a healthy gut environment. For heart health, polyphenols can help lower blood pressure and improve cardiovascular health by expanding blood vessels and preventing blood clots. They may also enhance brain function and protect against neurodegenerative diseases, according to some studies. Overall, including polyphenols in your diet can contribute to better health and well-being (45-47).

Berries: Blueberries, strawberries, and raspberries are packed with polyphenols that combat oxidative stress. They are like little power-packed grenades, exploding with goodness to rejuvenate your cells.

Dark Chocolate: Indulging in a square of dark chocolate is not just a treat—it is a luxurious spa day for your cells. Rich in polyphenols, dark chocolate helps reduce inflammation and improve heart health. So, go ahead, savor that square of chocolate—it is self-care for your body's defences

Green Tea: A cup of green tea is a ritual of relaxation and rejuvenation. Its polyphenols, particularly catechins, are excellent at mopping up free radicals and reducing oxidative stress. It is like a calming, cleansing wave for your cells.

Polyphenols are the unsung heroes of the antioxidant world, offering a host of health benefits that keep you feeling spry and vibrant.

Antioxidants in Action: Reducing Oxidative Stress and Promoting Health

Antioxidants work tirelessly to neutralize free radicals—those rogue molecules that can damage cells and contribute to aging and disease. By doing so, they help reduce oxidative stress and promote overall health. Here is how antioxidants make a difference:

Protecting Cells: Antioxidants protect cells from the damage caused by oxidative stress. This protection is crucial for maintaining healthy tissues and organs, from your skin to your heart.

Supporting Immune Function: A robust immune system is essential for defending against infections and diseases. Antioxidants like Vitamin C play a pivotal role in maintaining immune health.

Reducing Inflammation: Chronic inflammation is linked to numerous health conditions, including frailty. Antioxidants help reduce inflammation, supporting overall well-being and vitality.

Enhancing Skin Health: Vitamins A and E are particularly beneficial for skin health, helping to prevent damage from ultraviolet (UV) rays and other environmental stressors.

By incorporating a variety of antioxidant-rich foods into your diet, you are giving your body the tools it needs to fight oxidative stress and stay healthy.

Practical Tips for Boosting Your Antioxidant Intake

Incorporating more antioxidants into your diet does not have to be complicated. Here are some practical tips to get you started:

Eat the Rainbow: Include a variety of colorful fruits and vegetables in your meals. Each color represents different antioxidants, so the more colors, the better!

Snack Smart: Keep a stash of nuts and seeds for a quick and nutritious snack. They are rich in Vitamins E and A, offering a tasty way to boost your antioxidant intake.

Enjoy Berries: Add berries to your breakfast, whether in a smoothie, yogurt, or oatmeal. They are not only delicious but also packed with polyphenols.

Sip Green Tea: Swap out your usual beverage for a cup of green tea. It is a simple and effective way to increase your antioxidant intake.

Indulge Wisely: Treat yourself to a small piece of dark chocolate. It is a delightful way to enjoy the benefits of polyphenols while satisfying your sweet tooth.

In brief, antioxidants are your body's dedicated cleanup crew, tirelessly working to reduce oxidative stress and support overall health. By embracing a diet rich in antioxidants, you are giving your body the best possible defense against the wear and tear of daily life. So, let us raise a glass of green tea to these unsung heroes and enjoy the benefits they bring!

4.4 Addressing Common Micronutrient Deficiencies

Now that we have met the key players in the micronutrient league, it is time to tackle the gaps. Micronutrient deficiencies are more common than you would think, especially in older adults (48). Think of it as a detective mission—identifying and addressing these deficiencies can make a world of difference. Let us delve into the details.

Vitamin D Deficiency: The Silent Epidemic

As we age, our skin becomes less efficient at producing Vitamin D. Combine that with limited sun exposure, and you have got a recipe for deficiency. Vitamin D is essential for bone health, immune function, and mood regulation. Without enough of it, you might feel like a car running on empty.

How to Spot It:

Frequent Infections: Vitamin D supports your immune system, so frequent colds could be a sign.

Bone Pain: Persistent pain might indicate weakening bones.

Fatigue and Mood Swings: Low energy and mood changes can also hint at a deficiency.

The Fix:

Sunlight: Spend a few minutes in the sun daily. Morning or late afternoon sun is best to avoid harmful UV rays.

Supplements: If sun exposure is limited, consider a Vitamin D supplement after consulting with your doctor.

Diet: Include Vitamin D-rich foods like fatty fish (salmon, mackerel), fortified dairy products, and egg yolks.

B12 Deficiency: The Hidden Saboteur

B12 deficiency often masquerades as fatigue or forgetfulness. This vitamin is vital for nerve function and red blood cell production. Without enough B12, you might feel like a balloon slowly losing air.

How to Spot It:

Tiredness: Constant fatigue despite adequate rest.

Memory Issues: Forgetfulness and difficulty concentrating.

Pale Skin: B12 is key for red blood cells, so deficiency might cause paleness.

The Fix:

Blood Test: If you suspect you are low, ask your doctor about a blood test.

Fortified Foods: Consume B12-fortified cereals, nutritional yeast, and plant-based milks.

Supplements/Injections: In severe cases, B12 injections or high-dose supplements might be necessary. Your doctor will guide you on this.

Iron and Calcium: Balancing Act

Iron and calcium play a crucial role in keeping your body strong and healthy. Iron supports oxygen transport in your blood, while calcium is essential for bone health. However, they can interfere with each other's absorption, making timing everything.

How to Spot It:

Iron Deficiency: Look for fatigue, pale skin, and shortness of breath.

Calcium Deficiency: Noticeable signs include brittle nails, muscle cramps, and tooth decay.

The Fix:

Separate Intake: Take iron and calcium at different times of the day to ensure both nutrients get their due.

Iron-Rich Foods: Include lean meats, beans, lentils, and spinach in your diet.

Calcium-Rich Foods: Consume dairy products, fortified plant milks, tofu, and leafy greens.

Making Nutrition Accessible

Eating a balanced diet does not have to be complicated. Stock up on colorful fruits, vegetables, nuts, and seeds. If cooking feels daunting, pre-chopped or frozen options are just as nutritious. Small changes add up to big benefits.

Tips to Simplify Nutrition:

Plan Ahead: Prepare meals in advance and freeze portions for easy access.

Mix and Match: Create colorful salads with a variety of fruits and vegetables.

Snack Smart: Keep nuts, seeds, and fruit on hand for quick, nutritious snacks.

Stay Hydrated: Drinking plenty of water aids in nutrient absorption and overall health.

Wrapping It Up

Micronutrients may be small, but their impact is monumental. By giving your body, the vitamins, minerals, and antioxidants it needs, you are not just fighting frailty—you are building resilience. So, let us celebrate these tiny powerhouses and make them a staple in every meal. Your future self will thank you for the investment in your health and well-being.

CHAPTER 5: MALNUTRITION AND FRAILTY

When it comes to frailty, malnutrition is like a persistent fog that hovers and obscures well-being. The two go hand in hand, feeding off each other in a vicious cycle. Frailty makes it hard to get the nutrients you need, and malnutrition weakens the body even further, leaving you more vulnerable. It is like trying to climb out of quicksand with a backpack full of rocks. But here is the good news: recognizing the problem is the first step to breaking the cycle. Let us dive into how we can identify, assess, and address malnutrition to build resilience.

5.1 Identifying Malnutrition In Frail Individuals

Malnutrition is not always obvious. It is not just about being thin or losing weight; sometimes, it is about what you are missing. Think of your body like a car. If you are not getting enough fuel—whether that is protein, vitamins, or other nutrients—you will sputter along, no matter how much you weigh. And just like a car that is running on fumes, a malnourished body can only go so far before it starts showing signs of wear and tear.

Clues to Watch For

Unexplained Weight Loss: Losing weight without trying is not just suspicious—it is a flashing neon warning sign. Imagine stepping on the scale and noticing the numbers dropping, even though you have been eating your usual meals. That kind of weight loss often signals something deeper at play, especially in frail individuals. It is your body's way of telling you that it is running on empty or burning through reserves it should not have to.

Fatigue: Running on empty leaves you feeling tired and sluggish. If getting through the day feels like wading through molasses, malnutrition might be to blame. Your body needs fuel to function, and when it is not getting enough, every task becomes an uphill battle. Even the simplest activities—like brushing your hair or walking to the mailbox—can feel like climbing Mount Everest.

Muscle Loss: Frailty's best ally, sarcopenia, thrives on malnutrition. Imagine a shadowy figure slipping into your house, silently taking away your most cherished belongings. That is sarcopenia—it sneaks in and robs you of your muscle mass, leaving you weaker and more vulnerable. Over time, this muscle loss can make it harder to stay active, leading to a vicious cycle of frailty and malnutrition.

Appetite Changes: If food seems about as appealing as cardboard, it is time to dig deeper. A dwindling appetite can be one of the earliest symptoms of malnutrition. It is not always about eating less on purpose; sometimes, food just does not taste as good, or you are dealing with dental issues or digestive problems that make eating a chore instead of a pleasure.

Nutrient Deficiency Symptoms: Think brittle nails, thinning hair, or even sudden mood swings. Your body is like a finely tuned orchestra, where every nutrient plays a critical role. When key players like iron, vitamin D, or vitamin B12 decide to take a break, the harmonious symphony that keeps you energized and healthy can quickly spiral into discord. But what exactly does that mean for you? Let us dive into the fascinating, sometimes quirky world of nutrient deficiencies and how they affect everything from your energy levels to your mental health.

The Hair and Nail Chronicles: Signs You Can not Ignore

Ever noticed your nails looking like they have been through a battle? Maybe they are brittle, split easily, or have peculiar white spots. These are often telltale signs that your body's nutrient supply is running low. For instance, a lack of biotin—often referred to as the "beauty vitamin"—can leave your nails fragile and your hair lacklustre. Iron deficiency, on the other hand, can cause hair to thin and even fall out. Think of iron as the VIP ticket for oxygen to travel through your blood and nourish your hair follicles. Without it, your strands simply Can not party.

Energy Drain: When You Feel Like a Dying Phone Battery

If you constantly feel like you need a nap—even after a full night's sleep—you might be dealing with a nutrient deficiency. Low levels of vitamin B12 or iron can sap your energy because they are crucial for producing red blood cells, which ferry oxygen to your muscles and organs. It is like running a marathon with a backpack full of rocks. Not ideal, right?

Vitamin D, the so-called "sunshine vitamin," also deserves a shoutout here. It not only helps your bones stay strong but also plays a surprising role in keeping fatigue at bay. If you are skipping out on sunlight or not eating enough vitamin D-rich foods like fatty fish, your energy reserves could plummet faster than you think.

Immune System SOS: Why You are Always Sniffly

Your immune system is like the body's personal security detail, and it is fuelled by an intricate cocktail of vitamins and minerals. When key nutrients like vitamin C, zinc, or selenium are in short supply, your body's defences weaken. Suddenly, that harmless office cold turns into a full-blown, week-long misery. Vitamin C acts as a bodyguard for your cells, fighting off harmful invaders. Zinc, meanwhile, is the ultimate multitasker, helping your body heal wounds and fend off infections. If your immune system feels like it is constantly calling in sick, it might be time to reassess your diet.

Mood Swings and Mental Health: More Than Just a "Bad Day"

Feeling unusually down or irritable? Nutrient deficiencies could be messing with your brain's chemistry. Omega-3 fatty acids, for example, are vital for maintaining healthy brain function, and their deficiency can make you feel foggy or even anxious. Similarly, a shortage of magnesium—often called nature's relaxant—can make you more prone to stress and poor sleep.

Vitamin B12 and folate (vitamin B9) are also brain-health superstars. They are involved in producing neurotransmitters like serotonin and dopamine, which are your feel-good chemicals. When these vitamins are lacking, your mental health might take a nosedive, leaving you feeling like you have lost your spark.

Skin Deep: The Complexion Connection

Your skin is essentially a billboard advertising your internal health. Dryness, acne, or slow-healing wounds can all point to nutrient imbalances. Vitamin A keeps your skin smooth and vibrant, while zinc helps repair damage and prevent breakouts. Collagen production—key for firm, youthful skin—depends on vitamin C. So, if your skin is throwing tantrums, your diet might need some tweaking.

Gut Feelings: Digestion and Nutrient Deficiencies

Ever had that "off" feeling in your stomach? Nutrient deficiencies could be partly to blame. Ironically, a poor diet can create a vicious cycle: deficiencies can lead to digestive problems, and digestive problems can make it harder to absorb nutrients. For example, insufficient fiber intake can slow down digestion, while a lack of magnesium might contribute to bloating or constipation. Even your gut bacteria—which thrive on a diverse range of foods—can become less effective at breaking down food when nutrients are scarce.

Your body's nutrient needs are like the strings of a violin: delicate, intricate, and vital for the perfect tune. When one string is out of sync, the whole melody suffers. Pay attention to the clues—whether it is fatigue, brittle nails, or mood swings—and give your body the nutrients it needs to perform at its best. After all, life is too short to live out of tune.

Why Frailty Makes It Tricky

Frailty can make identifying malnutrition challenging. It is a master of disguise, often hiding behind other issues like fatigue, mobility challenges, or chronic illnesses. Appetite changes, chewing difficulties, and even depression can mask or exacerbate malnutrition. For example, someone who is struggling with arthritis might find it hard to prepare meals, while another person might avoid eating because of painful dentures. And then there is the emotional toll. Depression, loneliness, and anxiety can all take a bite out of your appetite, making it even harder to get the nutrients you need. The result? A downward spiral where malnutrition worsens frailty, and frailty makes malnutrition harder to spot.

The Importance of Early Detection

That is why early detection is key. If you suspect malnutrition, do not just guess—assess. Talk to your doctor, a dietitian, or another healthcare professional who can help pinpoint the problem and develop a plan to address it. Remember, malnutrition is not a one-size-fits-all issue. It is a puzzle with many pieces, and finding the right solution often requires a team effort.

So, if you or someone you love is showing indicators of malnutrition, do not wait. Take action. Because when it comes to frailty and malnutrition, the sooner you intervene, the better the chances of turning things around.

5.2 Consequences Of Malnutrition

Malnutrition is not just about feeling hungry or looking frail; it is like a silent saboteur, quietly wreaking havoc on your body and mind. Imagine an orchestra where every instrument is out of tune. That is your body on malnutrition—a symphony of problems, each one compounding the next. Let us break it down and explore how malnutrition affects both physical and cognitive health.

Physical Health: The Obvious and the Sneaky

Your body is a machine, and food is the fuel. But what happens when you run on empty? The answer is a cascade of physical problems, ranging from the ones you might expect to those that catch you off guard.

Weakness and Fatigue

Ever tried to drive a car with an empty gas tank? That is your body without proper nutrition. Without enough calories and essential nutrients, your muscles lose strength, and your energy reserves deplete faster than a smartphone battery on a busy day. This is not just about feeling tired; it is about struggling to climb stairs, carry groceries, or even stand for extended periods.

Delayed Healing

Have you ever wondered why that paper cut from last week still has not healed? Malnutrition slows down your body's repair system. Protein, vitamins, and minerals are the building blocks for tissue repair, and without them, wounds linger like unwanted houseguests. This is particularly dangerous for older adults or those with chronic illnesses, where even minor injuries can escalate into serious complications.

Increased Falls

Here is the sneaky part: malnutrition does not just weaken your muscles; it also messes with your balance. Poor nutrition affects the inner ear and muscles that help you stay upright. Combine that with brittle bones from nutrient deficiencies like calcium and vitamin D, and you have got a recipe for falls that are not only frequent but also potentially life-threatening.

Immune Suppression

Think of your immune system as your body's personal army. Without proper nutrition, this army is underfed and underprepared, making it harder to fight off invaders like bacteria and viruses. What does that mean for you? More colds, longer recoveries, and a higher risk of infections spiraling out of control.

Hidden Physical Costs

Malnutrition does not just stop at the surface. Inside, it is causing havoc too. Poor nutrition can lead to organ dysfunction, including a weakened heart and impaired kidney function. Even your digestive system suffers, as malnutrition reduces the production of essential enzymes needed to break down food, creating a vicious cycle of nutrient absorption issues.

Cognitive Health: Food for Thought

Your brain is a demanding diva, constantly requiring a steady stream of nutrients to keep the show running. When malnutrition sets in, the brain does not just whisper its complaints—it shouts them. Here is how your cognitive health takes a hit:

Memory Loss: If you have ever found yourself walking into a room and forgetting why you went there, malnutrition might be partly to blame. The brain's ability to form and retrieve memories depends on nutrients like omega-3 fatty acids, B vitamins, and glucose. Without these, your mental Rolodex starts losing cards, making even simple tasks frustrating.

Mood Changes: Feeling irritable, anxious, or downright blue? Your diet might have something to do with it. Nutrient deficiencies disrupt the production of neurotransmitters like serotonin and dopamine, which are essential for mood regulation. Think of it this way:

without the right ingredients, your brain's "happy chemicals" cannot cook up the feel-good vibes you need.

Cognitive Decline

Poor nutrition is not just a short-term problem; it is a long-term threat. Studies link malnutrition to an increased risk of dementia and other cognitive disorders. The brain's cells are highly sensitive to oxidative stress and inflammation, both of which are exacerbated by poor nutrition. Over time, this can lead to a decline in memory, problem-solving skills, and even personality changes.

The Domino Effect

When your brain struggles, so does the rest of you. Cognitive impairment can lead to poor decision-making, including the ability to maintain a healthy diet, creating a vicious cycle. It is a feedback loop where malnutrition feeds cognitive decline, and cognitive decline perpetuates malnutrition.

Why Malnutrition Does not Play Favorites

Malnutrition does not discriminate based on age, gender, or lifestyle. Whether you are young or old, active or sedentary, its effects can creep into your life. Older adults are particularly at risk due to factors like reduced appetite, difficulty chewing or swallowing, and social isolation. But the good news? Even small dietary changes can yield big benefits.

Turning the Tide: Small Changes, Big Impact

The solution to malnutrition is not a complicated formula; it is about making informed, sustainable choices. Adding nutrient-dense foods like fruits, vegetables, lean proteins, and whole grains to your diet can kickstart your body's healing processes and fuel your brain. For those struggling with appetite, nutrient-dense snacks or meal supplements can make a significant difference.

Final Thoughts

Malnutrition may be a silent attacker, but it is not undefeatable. Understanding its consequences on both physical and cognitive health is the first step toward combating it. With the right nutritional strategies, you can restore balance to your body and mind, reclaiming energy, strength, and mental clarity.

5.3 Assessment Tools For Malnutrition And Frailty

Imagine trying to fix a leaky faucet without knowing where the drip is coming from—frustrating, right? The same principle applies to malnutrition and frailty. These conditions often hide in plain sight, and to address them effectively, you first need to uncover the full picture. That is where screening and assessment tools come in, acting like a plumber's flashlight to illuminate the problem areas. Let us delve into the essential tools, timing, and role of healthcare providers in identifying these silent saboteurs of health.

Tools of the Trade

The Malnutrition Universal Screening Tool (MUST): MUST is a five-step screening tool to identify adults, who are malnourished, at risk of malnutrition (undernutrition), or obese. Picture this: a quick and straightforward tool that evaluates risk based on three factors—Body Mass Index (BMI), unintentional weight loss, and the impact of acute illness on nutritional intake. The MUST tool is like the Swiss Army knife of malnutrition screening—simple yet incredibly versatile. It is often the first step in identifying those at risk, whether they are at home, in a hospital, or part of a community program. It also includes management guidelines which can be used to develop a care plan.

Mini Nutritional Assessment (MNA): This tool was designed with older adults in mind—because who knows better about nutritional needs than the age group that is perfected the art of sneaking cookies from grandkids? The MNA goes beyond BMI, looking at dietary habits, weight changes, and even psychological stress, giving a holistic view of an individual's nutritional health. It is like having a conversation with your wise grandmother, only this one provides actionable insights.

Clinical Tests: Screening does not stop with questionnaires and scorecards. Blood tests can reveal deficiencies in key nutrients like iron, vitamin D, and B12, while muscle strength assessments (such as grip strength) and bone density scans give insights into physical resilience. These tests act as the laboratory detectives, uncovering clues that might not be obvious in daily life.

When and Where to Screen

Screening is not a one-time event—it is more like keeping tabs on the wear and tear of your favorite pair of shoes. Regular assessments are crucial, especially for older adults, individuals with chronic illnesses, or those recovering from surgery. Screening often starts in primary care clinics, where your trusted doctor might notice subtle red flags like unintended weight loss or fatigue. Hospitals, rehabilitation centers, and even community health programs are also hubs for identifying malnutrition and frailty. Community centers often host wellness fairs or health check-up camps, providing a less intimidating environment for initial screenings. Picture it as a pop-up detective agency dedicated to solving the mystery of hidden health risks.

The Role of Healthcare Providers

Healthcare providers are the Sherlock Holmes of the health world, armed with a keen eye for spotting the subtle signs of malnutrition and frailty. They rely on their clinical judgment, often corroborated by screening tools, to paint a complete picture of a patient's health. These experts know that frailty is not just about being physically weak—it is a complex interplay of physical, nutritional, and psychological factors.

So, if you have noticed something amiss—a loved one skipping meals, dropping weight, or struggling with daily activities—do not brush it off. Your healthcare provider is there to connect the dots, ask the right questions, and recommend the next steps. This is one scenario where being proactive is not just wise—it could be life-changing. Screening and assessment tools might not sound glamorous, but they are indispensable for ensuring healthy aging. By catching issues early and taking action, you are not just addressing a problem—you are paving the way for a brighter, healthier future.

Measuring Frailty in Older Adults

We have already mentioned different types of frailty tools in Chapter 1. Several tools and scales are used to assess frailty, each with its unique approach. These are mentioned again in brief here:

Fried Frailty Phenotype (FFP): Developed by Linda P. Fried and colleagues, this phenotype defines frailty as a clinical syndrome characterized by the presence of three or more of the following criteria: unintentional weight loss, self-reported exhaustion, weakness (grip strength), slow walking speed, and low physical activity. Individuals meeting three or more criteria are classified as frail, one or two as pre-frail, and none as non-frail (1).

Frailty Index (FI): The Frailty Index, also known as the Rockwood-Mitnitski Frailty Index, quantifies frailty by calculating the proportion of accumulated health deficits. It involves a comprehensive assessment of various deficits, including physical, cognitive, and nutritional factors (2). A higher index score indicates greater frailty, with scores above 0.21 or 0.25 typically indicating frailty.

Clinical Frailty Scale (CFS): The Clinical Frailty Scale, developed by Kenneth Rockwood and colleagues, is a judgment-based tool that assesses frailty based on clinical observations and patient history. It ranges from 1 (very fit) to 9 (terminally ill), with scores of 5 or higher indicating frailty (4). The CFS is easy to use and provides a quick assessment of an individual's overall health status.

Other Tools (5)

Edmonton Frail Scale: This scale evaluates nine domains, including cognition, general health, functional independence, social support, medication use, nutrition, mood, continence, and functional performance.

FRAIL Scale: A simple five-item questionnaire assessing fatigue, resistance, ambulation, illnesses, and loss of weight. It is quick to administer and useful in identifying frailty in clinical settings.

Timed Up-and-Go (TUG) Test: Measures the time it takes for an individual to stand up from a chair, walk three meters, turn around, and sit back down. Longer times indicate higher frailty risk.

Groningen Frailty Indicator (GFI): Assesses physical, cognitive, social, and psychological domains to identify frailty in community-dwelling elderly individuals.

Identification of Seniors at Risk (ISAR): A simple tool used in emergency departments to identify older adults at risk of adverse health outcomes.

Prisma-7: A seven-item questionnaire designed to screen for frailty in primary care settings, focusing on mobility, age, and health issues.

Survey of Health, Ageing and Retirement in Europe-Frailty Instrument (SHARE-FI): Combines self-reported data with objective measures to assess frailty in European populations.

Tilburg Frailty Indicator (TFI): Evaluates physical, psychological, and social frailty through a comprehensive questionnaire.

There are many other tools available for assessing frailty in different settings. All the tools are not suitable for common clinical uses. However, detailed description of all the tools are beyond the scope of this book. These tools provide valuable insights into the frailty status of older adults, helping healthcare professionals tailor interventions and improve patient outcomes.

5.4 Strategies To Address And Reverse Malnutrition

Now for the good stuff: reversing malnutrition and breaking the cycle of frailty. It is not rocket science, but it does take a mix of strategy, support, and persistence. With the right approach, even the most daunting health challenges can be tackled one bite at a time.

Nutritional Interventions

Protein Power: Protein is your muscle's best friend, and not all heroes wear capes—some come in the form of eggs, lean meats, beans, or tofu. Protein provides the essential building blocks for repairing and maintaining muscle mass, which is often the first casualty of malnutrition and frailty. If you are not keen on a steak dinner, try alternatives like yogurt, cheese, or even protein-enriched smoothies. The key is consistency—your muscles will thank you for every bite.

Micronutrient Marvels: While protein steals the spotlight, vitamins and minerals play an equally starring role. Vitamins D and B12, calcium, and iron often need extra attention as we age. Vitamin D is like the sunshine nutrient, essential for bone health and immune function. Meanwhile, B12 keeps your nerve and blood cells in tip-top shape. Calcium ensures those bones stay strong, and iron carries oxygen to every corner of your body. Incorporating fortified foods, supplements, or naturally rich sources like leafy greens, fish, and dairy can make a world of difference.

Small, Frequent Meals: If the thought of a large meal feels overwhelming, think snack-sized. Smaller, frequent meals can make it easier to keep up with nutritional needs without the pressure of a full plate. It is like grazing at a buffet—only this time, you are focusing on nutrient-dense options like nuts, fruits, and whole-grain crackers.

Fortified Foods: Sometimes, nature needs a little help from science. Fortified cereals, drinks, and even snack bars can fill in the nutritional gaps, especially when appetite or dietary restrictions limit natural food choices. Think of them as your nutritional safety net—there when you need them.

Practical Tips

Meal Planning: Planning meals does not have to be a chore; it can be an adventure. Imagine designing a menu that is as exciting as planning a vacation—picking colorful fruits, experimenting with new recipes, and creating balanced plates that look as good as they taste. A little foresight goes a long way in ensuring every meal counts.

Social Eating: Eating alone can feel like a solitary chore, but add a friend, family member, or community group, and meals become an event. Sharing food fosters connection and joy, making it easier to eat well and stick to healthy habits. Bonus points if the social element encourages you to try new dishes or recipes.

Texture Tweaks: For those with chewing or swallowing difficulties, texture can be a game-changer. Softer foods like mashed potatoes, stews, and thickened soups ensure meals are both nutritious and easy to consume. Do not shy away from experimenting—sometimes a blended smoothie or pureed dish can be just as satisfying as the original.

Hydration: Water might not seem glamorous, but it is a silent MVP in maintaining health. Dehydration can sneak up on anyone, especially older adults, leading to fatigue, confusion, and a host of other issues. Keep fluids varied and interesting with herbal teas, infused water, or broths to ensure hydration stays on track.

Beyond the Plate

Nutrition alone is not enough to reverse the effects of malnutrition and frailty. A holistic approach that incorporates physical, emotional, and social well-being is essential for long-term success.

Exercise: Movement is medicine. Even light activity, like stretching or a short walk, can stimulate appetite, improve circulation, and strengthen muscles. Tailor exercise to individual abilities—every little bit helps, and over time, small efforts can lead to big gains in strength and energy.

Emotional Support: Malnutrition often goes hand in hand with emotional challenges like depression, loneliness, or anxiety. Addressing these feelings can unlock the motivation to eat well and take care of oneself. Whether through therapy, support groups, or simply opening up to a trusted friend, emotional well-being is an essential ingredient in the recipe for recovery.

Healthcare Collaboration: When it comes to personalized care, healthcare providers are your best allies. Dietitians, doctors, and nutritionists can help craft tailored plans that address specific needs and preferences. Think of them as the architects of your health strategy—laying the foundation for a successful turnaround.

Celebrate Small Wins

Reversing malnutrition is not about achieving perfection overnight; it is about making steady, meaningful progress. Celebrate every small victory—whether it is finishing a nutritious meal, trying a new food, or regaining the energy to enjoy a favorite activity. These moments are the building blocks of resilience.

Malnutrition and frailty may seem like an unstoppable duo, but with awareness, tools, and strategies, they are challenges we can overcome. Every bite, every positive change, is a step toward rewriting the story of frailty. Let us build a future where health and vitality take center stage, one nourishing meal at a time.

CHAPTER 6: GUT AND FRAILTY LINK

Aging gracefully is an art, but when malnutrition and frailty team up, they can turn the golden years into a wobbly tightrope walk. Let us explore how our gut health, diet, and some helpful microbes take center stage in this balancing act.

6.1 How Gut Health Influences Frailty

Imagine your gut as a bustling city, teeming with trillions of microscopic residents—bacteria, viruses, fungi—all collectively known as the gut microbiome. This metropolis does not just digest your breakfast; it influences your immunity, mood, and yes, your muscle strength. As we age, the city's landscape changes, and not always for the better.

Studies have shown that as we age, the variety of friendly bacteria in our gut can decline, kind of like a once-bustling city losing some of its most vibrant neighborhoods. This lack of diversity in our gut microbiota can cause problems. One major issue is something called "leaky gut," where the gut lining becomes more permeable. Imagine your gut lining as a fine mesh sieve that lets through the good stuff but blocks the bad. When the mesh gets damaged, unwanted substances can slip through into the bloodstream, triggering long lingering inflammation. This chronic inflammation is a bit like a smouldering fire that never fully goes out. Over time, it can contribute to frailty, which is when your body becomes weaker and more vulnerable. One of the key ways this happens is through a loss of muscle mass and strength, a condition known as sarcopenia. Picture it as your muscles slowly shrinking and losing power, making everyday tasks harder and increasing the risk of falls and injuries. Recognizing the role of gut health in preventing frailty highlights the importance of a balanced diet and lifestyle to maintain a diverse and healthy gut microbiota (49). There is a growing body of evidence supporting the importance of gut health and diet in overall well-being. Here are some key findings:

High-Fiber Diet: Studies have shown that a diet rich in fiber, including whole grains, fruits, vegetables, and legumes, promotes a healthy gut microbiome (50). Fiber acts as food for beneficial gut bacteria, helping them thrive and maintain a balanced ecosystem (51).

Fermented Foods: Fermented products, such as yogurt, kimchi, sauerkraut, miso, and kefir, are especially important. These foods undergo a natural fermentation process where friendly bacteria, like probiotics, grow and thrive (50). When you eat fermented foods, you are adding even more beneficial bacteria to your gut city. It is like bringing in reinforcements to your team of superheroes. These reinforcements help improve your digestion, boost your immune system, and enhance your overall vitality.

Gut Microbiome and Chronic Diseases: Research indicates that the gut microbiome plays a role in modulating the risk of chronic diseases such as obesity, type 2 diabetes mellitus, cardiovascular disease, and even certain cancers (51). A healthy gut microbiome can help reduce inflammation and improve metabolic health (51).

Resistant Starch: Foods high in resistant starch, such as beans, lentils, and whole grains, are particularly beneficial for gut health. Resistant starch is not digested in the small intestine and reaches the colon, where it feeds beneficial bacteria and promotes their growth (50).

Dietary Impact on Microbial Composition: Studies have shown that dietary changes can induce significant shifts in the gut microbiome within 24 hours. These shifts can have broad implications for health, including immune and metabolic functions (51).

But it is not all doom and gloom. The good news is that maintaining a diverse and balanced gut microbiome can be like having a trusty shield against frailty. Imagine your gut microbiome as a bustling city filled with different types of friendly bacteria. When this city is diverse and vibrant, it helps keep your body strong and healthy. Research has shown that individuals with a richer and more varied gut microbiota tend to have better physical function and are less prone to frailty (52). These bacteria work together to keep everything running smoothly and to protect you from getting sick. When you take care of your gut, you are not only helping your digestion but also boosting your overall health and energy levels. Each type of food brings in different bacteria that have unique skills and benefits. This diverse team helps create a well-functioning, resilient community that shields you from becoming frail or weak.

6.2 Impact Of Diet On Gut Microbiome In Older Adults

You are what you eat, and so are your gut microbes. Diet is a major architect of your gut's skyline. Fiber-rich foods, like fruits, vegetables, and whole grains, serve as prebiotics —essentially the gourmet meals for beneficial bacteria. Prebiotics are types of dietary fiber that serve as food for beneficial gut bacteria. Unlike probiotics, which are live bacteria, prebiotics are non-digestible food components that travel to the colon, where they are fermented by the gut microbiome. Think of prebiotics as the fuel that powers your superhero team of gut bacteria. Prebiotics selectively stimulate the growth and activity of beneficial bacteria in the gut. By providing the necessary nutrients for these good bacteria, prebiotics help maintain a balanced and healthy gut microbiome. This, in turn, supports various aspects of health, including improved digestion, enhanced immune function, and better absorption of nutrients. On the flip side, a diet high in processed foods and low in fiber can lead to a decline in microbial diversity.

Imagine a diet that is like a Mediterranean vacation for your gut—colorful, flavourful, and full of health benefits. A Mediterranean diet, rich in fruits, vegetables, legumes, and olive oil, has been associated with fantastic changes in the gut microbiome, the bustling community of bacteria living in your digestive system.

Here is the scoop: A study involving older adults found that those who followed a Mediterranean diet for a year experienced significant improvements in their gut health. This was not just about feeling good after a meal; these beneficial changes in their microbiome were linked to reduced frailty and better overall health (13). The Mediterranean diet is a feast for your senses and your cells. It is packed with fresh fruits and vegetables that provide essential vitamins and minerals, legumes like beans and lentils that offer protein and fiber, and olive oil, which is rich in healthy fats. These foods work together to nourish your body and support a diverse and balanced gut microbiome.

Think of your gut microbiome as a garden. The Mediterranean diet is like the perfect fertilizer, helping good bacteria thrive and keeping harmful ones at bay. This balance is crucial because a healthy gut can reduce inflammation, improve digestion, and boost your immune system.

In the study, the participants who stuck to the Mediterranean diet showed fewer signs of frailty. They had better physical function, which means they could move around more easily and had stronger muscles. Plus, their overall health improved, making them feel more energetic and resilient.

So, if you are looking for a way to support your health and keep frailty at bay, the Mediterranean diet might be your answer. It is not just a diet; it is a lifestyle that celebrates fresh, wholesome foods and mindful eating. Whether you are savouring a vibrant salad, enjoying a hearty bowl of lentil soup, or drizzling olive oil over roasted veggies, you are giving your gut the love and care it needs to keep you strong and healthy.

But it is not just about what you eat; it is also about what you do not eat. Overindulging in red meat and high-fat foods can be like throwing a wild party for the wrong crowd in your gut. These foods can promote the growth of harmful bacteria, which in turn can lead to inflammation. Think of inflammation as your body's internal fire alarm—it goes off when there is trouble, and too much of it can lead to serious health issues, including cancer (53, 54).

Moderation is key here. Enjoying a steak or a burger now and then is not going to ruin your health, but making it a daily habit might. It is like trying to balance on a seesaw; too much weight on one side, and things start to tip over. The goal is to find that sweet spot where you are not overloading on the bad stuff.

Incorporating a variety of plant-based foods into your diet can help maintain a balanced gut microbiome. These foods are like the VIPs you want at your gut party—think colorful vegetables, fruits, legumes, nuts, and seeds. They bring fiber, vitamins, and antioxidants to the table, which help keep your gut bacteria diverse and thriving.

Eating plant-based foods can be delicious and fun. Imagine a vibrant salad with a rainbow of veggies, a hearty bean stew, or a refreshing fruit smoothie. These foods not only taste great but also support your gut health, making your microbiome a well-oiled machine. So, the next time you are planning a meal, think about the balance. It is okay to enjoy a little red meat or a rich dessert, but make sure you are also inviting plenty of plant-based foods to the party. Your gut—and your whole body—will thank you for it.

6.3 Probiotics, Prebiotics, And Their Role In Resilience

Previously touched upon, let us delve into the details of the dynamic duo for your gut: probiotics and prebiotics. Imagine probiotics as the good guys—the live beneficial bacteria that help keep your gut healthy. You can find these friendly bacteria in foods like yogurt, kefir, sauerkraut, and other fermented products. They work tirelessly to maintain a balanced gut microbiome, which is necessary for your overall health and resilience. On the other hand, prebiotics are like the fuel for these good bacteria. They are non-digestible fibers found in foods such as garlic, onions, bananas, and asparagus. Prebiotics serve as food for probiotics, helping them flourish and do their job more effectively. Think of prebiotics as the fertilizer that helps your garden of probiotics grow strong and healthy.

When probiotics and prebiotics team up, they can significantly enhance your gut health, which in turn boosts your overall resilience. This powerful partnership can be especially beneficial for older adults, who often face challenges related to gut health and frailty. Studies have shown that supplementing with probiotics can lead to improvements in muscle strength and physical performance in older adults. A review found that probiotic supplementation not only improved muscle strength but also suggested a positive effect on muscle mass (55). This means that incorporating probiotics into your diet could help keep your muscles strong and your body agile as you age.

But what about prebiotics? Prebiotics, found in foods like garlic, onions, and bananas, can also play a role. They promote the growth of beneficial bacteria, which in turn produce short-chain fatty acids that have anti-inflammatory properties. This anti-inflammatory effect can help mitigate the chronic inflammation associated with frailty. Imagine them as tiny firefighters, constantly working to put out the flames of inflammation in your body. It is important to note that while the benefits of probiotics and prebiotics are promising, we still have a lot to learn. More research is needed to determine the optimal types and dosages for preventing or treating frailty (56).

6.4 Emerging Research On Gut-Brain-Muscle Connections

The plot thickens with the gut-brain-muscle axis—a fascinating and complex communication network where your gut microbiome, brain, and muscles are in constant conversation. Imagine this network as a lively group chat where everyone shares emojis and updates about your health status. This ongoing communication is crucial for maintaining overall well-being.

Emerging research has shed light on how the gut microbiota—the community of bacteria living in your digestive system—can influence muscle function and cognitive behavior. These tiny microbes play a much bigger role in our health than we might have imagined. Alterations in the composition of gut microbiota have been linked to changes in muscle physiology and cognitive function. This means that an imbalance in your gut bacteria could potentially impact muscle strength and mental sharpness, hinting at a role in conditions like sarcopenia (loss of muscle mass and strength) and cognitive decline (57). Let us break this down further:

The Gut-Brain Connection: Your gut and brain are in constant communication through a system known as the gut-brain axis. This connection involves multiple pathways, including the vagus nerve, hormones, and immune system signals. Essentially, your gut can send messages to your brain, and vice versa. This means that the health of your gut microbiome can influence your mood, stress levels, and cognitive functions. For example, certain gut bacteria produce neurotransmitters like serotonin and dopamine, which are crucial for regulating mood and cognition. An imbalance in these bacteria can disrupt these chemical signals, potentially leading to issues like anxiety, depression, or cognitive decline.

The Gut-Muscle Connection: Similarly, the gut-muscle axis highlights the relationship between gut health and muscle function. Beneficial bacteria in your gut produce short-chain fatty acids (SCFAs) when they ferment dietary fibers. These SCFAs have anti-inflammatory properties and can support muscle health. They help reduce inflammation in the body, which is particularly important for maintaining muscle mass and strength as we age.

Research has shown that a healthy and diverse gut microbiome can promote better muscle function. On the flip side, an imbalance in gut bacteria—often caused by poor diet, stress, or illness—can lead to increased inflammation and muscle wasting. Imagine your gut bacteria as the personal trainers for your muscles, guiding them to stay strong and resilient.

The Vicious Cycle of Imbalance

When your gut microbiota becomes imbalanced, it can set off a chain reaction that affects both the brain and muscles. This imbalance can increase gut permeability, sometimes referred to as "leaky gut." When the gut barrier becomes more permeable, it allows unwanted substances to enter the bloodstream, triggering inflammation throughout the body. Chronic inflammation is a key player in the development of frailty, making it harder to maintain muscle mass and cognitive function.

Moreover, the gut-brain axis, a bidirectional communication system between the gut and the brain, plays a crucial role in maintaining homeostasis. Disruptions in this axis have been associated with various neurodegenerative diseases, highlighting the importance of gut health in maintaining cognitive function (58). To understand this you need to delve a bit deeper into the fascinating world of the gut-brain axis—an incredible communication system that works both ways between your gut and your brain. Imagine it as a high-speed internet connection, constantly sending and receiving messages to keep everything running smoothly and in balance. This communication network is crucial for maintaining homeostasis, which is just a fancy term for your body's ability to keep its internal environment stable and healthy.

But what happens when this communication system gets disrupted? Well, things can go a bit haywire. Disruptions in the gut-brain axis have been linked to a range of neurodegenerative diseases, such as Alzheimer's disease and Parkinson's disease. These diseases can profoundly impact cognitive function, leading to issues with memory, thinking, and movement. This connection highlights just how important gut health is for maintaining not just your physical health, but also your brain function. Let us break it down further:

The Gut: Your Second Brain

Your gut is often referred to as your "second brain" because it has its own nervous system, known as the enteric nervous system. This system contains millions of neurons that communicate directly with your brain. Think of it as a mini-brain that oversees everything happening in your digestive system and beyond.

The Brain: Command Central

Your brain, the control center of your body, relies heavily on signals from the gut. This connection affects your mood, stress levels, and overall cognitive function. It is like having a smart assistant that alerts you when something's off balance, ensuring you stay in optimal health.

Communication Breakdown

When the gut-brain axis functions smoothly, it helps keep your body in harmony. However, when this communication system breaks down, it can lead to a host of problems. For example, an imbalance in your gut microbiome—an assortment of bacteria living in your digestive tract—can send distress signals to your brain. This can trigger inflammation and stress responses that impact your brain's health and function.

The Role of Gut Health in Cognitive Function

Maintaining a healthy gut microbiome is essential for supporting cognitive function. Your gut produces neurotransmitters like serotonin and dopamine, which are critical for mood regulation and mental clarity. When your gut microbiome is in good shape, it helps ensure that these neurotransmitters are produced in the right amounts, keeping you feeling mentally sharp and emotionally balanced.

The Impact of Neurodegenerative Diseases

Neurodegenerative diseases like Alzheimer's disease and Parkinson's disease are characterized by the gradual degeneration of neurons in the brain. Studies have shown that disruptions in the gut-brain axis can contribute to the development and progression of these diseases (59-61). For instance, chronic inflammation originating from the gut can accelerate neuronal damage and cognitive decline.

Practical Steps to Support the Gut-Brain-Muscle Axis

The good news is that you can start incorporating these gut-friendly foods into your diet right away. So, how can you support this vital communication network and maintain a healthy gut-brain-muscle axis? Here are some practical tips:

Add Probiotic-Rich Foods: Start your day with a serving of yogurt or kefir. These fermented dairy products are loaded with probiotics. You can also try adding sauerkraut or kimchi to your meals for an extra probiotic boost.

Include Prebiotic Foods: Make sure to include prebiotic-rich foods in your diet. Toss some bananas into your morning smoothie, add garlic and onions to your dishes, and snack on a handful of nuts.

Mix and Match: Combine probiotic and prebiotic foods for maximum benefit. For example, a yogurt parfait with bananas and a drizzle of honey is a delicious and gut-friendly treat.

Stay Consistent: Regularly consuming these foods can help maintain a healthy balance of gut bacteria. Make them a staple in your daily diet to support long-term gut health.

Consider Supplements: If you find it challenging to get enough probiotics and prebiotics from food alone, you might consider supplements. Always consult with a healthcare provider before starting any new supplement regimen.

Incorporating probiotics and prebiotics into your diet is like giving your gut a VIP treatment. By nurturing your gut microbiome, you are not just supporting digestion but also enhancing your overall health and resilience. So, why not give your gut the love it deserves? Your future self will thank you for it.

CHAPTER 7: PRACTICAL NUTRITION STRATEGIES FOR FRAIL ADULTS

Embarking on the journey of aging does not mean leaving behind the joys of good food. With the right nutritional compass, frail adults also can navigate their way to enhanced vitality and resilience. Let us dive into some practical, and dare we say, delightful strategies to make nutrition not just a necessity, but a pleasure.

7.1 Meal Planning And Preparation Tips

Imagine meal planning as crafting a symphony, where each ingredient plays its part in creating a harmonious and health-boosting melody. For frail individuals, this symphony should focus on nutrient-dense foods that are as rich in flavor as they are in benefits.

The Art of Simplicity

Keep recipes straightforward. Think of dishes that require minimal preparation but offer maximum nutrition. For instance, a hearty bowl of oatmeal topped with fresh berries and a sprinkle of nuts provides fiber, vitamins, and healthy fats without the need for a culinary degree (62).

Embracing Nutrient-Dense Ingredients

Incorporate foods that pack a nutritional punch in every bite. Leafy greens like spinach and kale are excellent sources of vitamins A, C, and K, as well as folate and iron. Adding a handful to soups, stews, or smoothies can enhance both flavor and health benefits. Similarly, fatty fish such as salmon provides omega-3 fatty acids, which are essential for heart health. A simple baked salmon with a side of steamed broccoli and sweet potatoes offers a meal rich in nutrients and flavor.

Prioritizing Protein

Protein is vital for maintaining muscle mass, especially in frail individuals. Incorporate lean meats, legumes, and dairy into meals. For example, a lentil soup not only warms the soul but also delivers a substantial amount of protein and fiber. Additionally, eggs are a versatile and easy-to-prepare protein source; a vegetable omelette can be both nutritious and satisfying. Include lean proteins like chicken, fish, or plant-based options such as beans and lentils.

These not only support muscle health but also keep energy levels steady throughout the day (23).

Incorporating Healthy Fats

Healthy fats are crucial for overall well-being. Avocado, nuts, and olive oil are excellent sources. A simple avocado toast sprinkled with chia seeds can serve as a quick, nutrient-dense meal or snack. Drizzling olive oil over roasted vegetables not only enhances flavor but also provides beneficial monounsaturated fats.

Color Your Plate

A vibrant plate is not just Instagram-worthy; it is a sign of a well-balanced meal. Incorporate a rainbow of fruits and vegetables to ensure a variety of nutrients. Carrots, spinach, blueberries, and tomatoes each bring their own unique health benefits to the table (63).

Hydration Station

Do not let dehydration sneak up on you. Hydration is often overlooked but is essential for health. Soups and stews are excellent ways to increase fluid intake while providing nutrients. A minestrone soup, loaded with vegetables and beans, offers hydration, fiber, and protein in a single bowl. Herbal teas and infused waters can also encourage adequate fluid consumption throughout the day (64).

Adapting to Individual Needs

It is important to tailor meals to individual preferences and dietary restrictions. Some may require softer foods due to dental issues, while others might need to monitor sodium intake. Consulting with a healthcare professional or registered dietitian can provide personalized guidance to ensure nutritional needs are met effectively.

In summary, crafting a nutritional symphony for frail individuals involves selecting simple, nutrient-dense ingredients that are easy to prepare and tailored to individual needs. By focusing on these elements, meal planning can become a harmonious endeavor that promotes health and well-being.

7.2 Nutritional Supplementation

Ah, supplements—the sidekicks to our dietary superheroes. But even sidekicks need to know their role to be effective.

Assess the Need

Before reaching for that bottle of multivitamins, it is essential to determine what is actually needed. Over-supplementation can be as problematic as deficiencies (65). Consulting with a healthcare professional can provide clarity.

Protein Supplements

For those struggling to meet protein requirements through food alone, protein shakes or powders can be beneficial. However, they should complement the diet, not replace whole foods (66).

Vitamin D and Calcium

Bone health is paramount. While it is best to obtain nutrients from food, supplements can help fill the gaps, especially in individuals with limited sun exposure or dietary restrictions. Reducing the risk of fractures and falls in older adults is not as straightforward as just taking a supplement. The United States Preventive Services Task Force (USPSTF) recommends against supplementation with vitamin D with or without calcium for the primary prevention of fractures in community-dwelling postmenopausal women and men aged 60 years or older. If your vitamin D and calcium levels are already adequate, supplements would not make much difference in preventing falls or fractures. Supplements are only beneficial if you are deficient in these nutrients (67).

Timing Matters

Some supplements are best taken with meals to enhance absorption, while others might need to be consumed on an empty stomach. Reading labels and following recommendations can make a significant difference (65).

7.3 Overcoming Appetite Loss And Eating Difficulties

When the appetite dwindles, mealtime can feel more like a chore than a delight. But fear not, for there are strategies to reignite the joy of eating. There are many causes of appetite loss in older adults (68):

Dehydration is a common issue among older adults, often due to not drinking enough fluids, which can be caused by medications, forgetfulness, or a lack of thirst. Dehydration can lead to serious health problems like kidney stones, UTIs, and an increased risk of falls, and it can also reduce appetite.

Eating alone can feel very lonely, and some older adults might skip meals because they do not want to eat by themselves or prepare food just for one person. Depression, which affects up to 20% of older adults, can also cause a loss of appetite. If you notice signs of depression, such as sadness, lack of energy, or poor sleep habits, it is important to seek help.

Sometimes older adults feel like they have lost control over their lives, especially regarding meal choices, which can affect their appetite. Including them in meal planning and preparation can help them feel more in control.

Difficulty chewing or swallowing due to dental issues, medications, or medical conditions can make eating unpleasant. Blending foods into smoothies, taking smaller bites, and eating slowly can make mealtime easier.

A sedentary lifestyle can lead to a reduced appetite. Older adults should aim for 150 minutes of physical activity each week, which can be broken down into short intervals. This can include strength training, balance exercises, aerobic activities, and flexibility training.

Changes in diet or unfamiliar foods can also cause a loss of appetite. If a senior is served foods they do not like, they may not eat enough. Experimenting with different flavors and using healthy alternatives to sugar and salt can help if they experience a loss of taste, which can make food less appealing.

A reduced sense of smell, often caused by aging, can decrease the enjoyment of food. This can be accelerated by diseases, smoking, and exposure to harmful particles.

Lastly, without a regular eating schedule, older adults might skip meals. Establishing a routine with 5-6 small meals throughout the day can help them meet their nutritional needs and improve their overall health.

These factors can impact an older person's desire to eat, but with a few adjustments, their appetite can often be improved. If you or a loved one are facing these challenges, consider these tips to help maintain a healthy diet.

Small, Frequent Meals

Instead of three large meals, opt for smaller, more frequent ones. This approach can make eating less daunting and ensure a steady intake of nutrients (68).

Enhance Flavors

A diminished sense of taste can dampen appetite. Experiment with herbs and spices to make dishes more enticing. A dash of cinnamon in porridge or a sprinkle of basil on pasta can work wonders (69).

Social Dining

Sharing meals with others can transform eating into a social event rather than a solitary task. Whether it is family, friends, or community groups, companionship can boost appetite and mood (68). When we eat with family, friends, or community groups, the companionship not only makes the meal more enjoyable but also offers several benefits for our physical and emotional well-being.

Boosts Appetite: Companionship during meals can significantly enhance one's appetite. The presence of others often encourages us to eat more, especially if the conversation is engaging and the atmosphere is positive. This can be particularly beneficial for older adults who might struggle with a lack of appetite when dining alone. The social interaction acts as a natural stimulant, making the mealtime more appealing.

Enhances Mood: Eating with others can elevate our mood and reduce feelings of loneliness and isolation. Sharing stories, laughter, and conversations around the dining table fosters a sense of connection and belonging. This social bond can improve mental health, reduce stress, and even lower the risk of depression. The simple act of sharing a meal can transform our emotional state, making us feel more content and fulfilled.

Creates a Sense of Community: Participating in communal meals, whether with family, friends, or through community groups, strengthens social ties and builds a sense of community. These gatherings provide an opportunity to engage with others, share experiences, and create lasting memories. For older adults, community meal programs can be a lifeline, offering not just nutritious food but also a chance to interact and form new friendships.

Encourages Healthy Eating Habits: When we eat with others, we are more likely to make healthier food choices. The influence of peers can encourage us to try new foods, stick to portion sizes, and maintain a balanced diet. Additionally, preparing and sharing meals together can be a fun and educational experience, promoting healthier cooking practices and a greater appreciation for nutritious foods.

Supports Cultural Traditions: Sharing meals is an excellent way to preserve and celebrate cultural traditions. Family recipes and traditional dishes can be passed down through generations, keeping cultural heritage alive. These shared culinary experiences can deepen our connection to our roots and provide a sense of continuity and identity.

Texture Matters

For those with chewing or swallowing difficulties, consider softer food options or modifying textures. Smoothies, soups, and stews are both gentle on the palate and nutrient-rich (70).

7.4 Culturally Appropriate And Affordable Dietary Solutions

Food is a profound expression of cultural heritage and personal identity, playing a pivotal role in the well-being of older adults. Crafting dietary solutions that honour cultural preferences while remaining affordable can significantly enhance meal satisfaction and adherence to nutritional guidelines.

Embrace Traditional Foods

Incorporate familiar ingredients and recipes that resonate with cultural backgrounds. Familiar ingredients and recipes provide comfort and a sense of belonging, which is crucial for mental and emotional well-being (71). For instance, maintaining traditional eating habits has been linked to better mental health outcomes among older adults. Additionally, traditional diets often emphasize plant-based foods, lean proteins, and whole grains, contributing to overall health. The Okinawan diet, rich in vegetables and low in calories, is associated with longevity and reduced chronic disease risk.

Affordable Choices

Eating well does not have to break the bank. Seasonal produce, grains, and legumes are often cost-effective and versatile. Planning meals around these staples can be both economical and healthful (64). In fact, there are plenty of nutritious foods that are affordable and versatile. Seasonal produce is a great example. Fruits and vegetables that are in season are often cheaper because they are more abundant and do not require long-distance shipping. Plus, they are fresher and usually taste better. By shopping for seasonal produce, you can enjoy a variety of nutrients throughout the year without spending a fortune.

Grains and legumes are also cost-effective staples. Items like rice, oats, quinoa, lentils, beans, and chickpeas are not only inexpensive but also packed with essential nutrients like protein, fiber, vitamins, and minerals. They are incredibly versatile and can be used in a wide range of dishes, from soups and stews to salads and casseroles.

Meal planning around these staples can further stretch your food budget while ensuring you maintain a balanced diet. Start by selecting a few staple ingredients and then look for recipes that incorporate them. For example, you can buy a bag of lentils and use them in a lentil soup, a hearty stew, and a refreshing salad. Similarly, a bunch of seasonal vegetables can be roasted, added to pasta, or turned into a stir-fry. Additionally, buying in bulk can save money in the long run. Many grains and legumes have a long shelf life and can be stored easily, making bulk purchases both economical and convenient.

By focusing on these cost-effective and nutritious options, you can create a variety of delicious, healthy meals without breaking the bank. Not only will this approach benefit your wallet, but it will also support your overall health and well-being.

Community Resources

Many communities offer programs that provide culturally appropriate meals for older adults. Engaging with these resources can offer support and variety (15). These programs can significantly enhance the well-being of older adults by ensuring they have access to nutritious, familiar, and enjoyable meals. Here are some key aspects of these community resources:

Senior Centers and Community Centers: Senior centers and community centers often have meal programs specifically designed for older adults. These programs offer meals that cater to the cultural preferences and dietary requirements of the participants. By providing culturally appropriate meals, these centers help older adults maintain their cultural identity and enjoy the foods they love.

Meals on Wheels: Many local 'Meals on Wheels' programs have expanded their offerings to include culturally diverse meal options. These programs deliver hot, nutritious meals directly to the homes of older adults who may have difficulty preparing food themselves. By offering culturally appropriate meals, 'Meals on Wheels' ensures that older adults can enjoy familiar flavors and dishes while receiving the nutrition they need.

Faith-Based Organizations: Churches, mosques, temples, and other faith-based organizations often run meal programs for their communities. These programs typically offer meals that align with the dietary practices and cultural preferences of their members. Engaging with these resources can provide older adults with a sense of community and belonging while enjoying meals that are meaningful to them.

Ethnic Community Groups: Many ethnic community groups organize meal programs and social events for older adults within their communities. These groups often focus on preserving and celebrating cultural traditions, including traditional cuisine. Participating in these programs can offer older adults a sense of connection and continuity with their cultural heritage.

Food Banks and Pantries: Some food banks and pantries offer culturally appropriate food items as part of their services. These organizations work to provide diverse food options to meet the needs of their clients. By accessing these resources, older adults can find ingredients and products that align with their cultural dietary practices.

Community Gardens: Community gardens can be a valuable resource for older adults looking to grow their own culturally significant foods. These gardens provide a space for individuals to cultivate fruits, vegetables, and herbs that are essential to their traditional diets. Engaging in community gardening can also promote physical activity and social interaction.

By engaging with these community resources, older adults can enjoy a variety of nutritious and culturally appropriate meals. These programs not only support their physical health but also contribute to their overall well-being by fostering a sense of community and cultural continuity.

Spice of Life

Utilize traditional herbs and spices not only for flavor but also for their potential health benefits. Herbs and spices have been used for centuries to enhance the flavor of food, but they also offer a variety of health benefits. Turmeric, garlic, and ginger, for example, are staples in many cultures and pack a nutritional punch (69). Incorporating these traditional ingredients into your diet can add a delightful twist to your meals while boosting your overall health. Here are a few examples:

Turmeric: Turmeric is a vibrant yellow spice commonly used in Indian, Pakistani, Bangladeshi, Southeast Asian, and Middle Eastern cuisine. It is known for its anti-inflammatory and antioxidant properties, thanks to a compound called curcumin. Incorporating turmeric into your diet can help reduce inflammation, improve brain function, and even lower the risk of chronic diseases. You can add it to curries, soups, smoothies, and teas for a flavourful and healthful boost.

Garlic: Garlic is a staple in many culinary traditions around the world. It is not only cherished for its pungent flavor but also for its numerous health benefits. Garlic contains allicin, a compound with potent medicinal properties. Regular consumption of garlic can help lower blood pressure, reduce cholesterol levels, and boost the immune system. Use garlic in sautés, marinades, sauces, and dressings to reap its benefits.

Ginger: Ginger is another powerful spice with a long history of use in traditional medicine. It is well-known for its anti-inflammatory and antioxidant effects. Ginger can help alleviate nausea, improve digestion, and reduce muscle pain and soreness. You can incorporate ginger into your diet by adding it to stir-fries, soups, smoothies, and teas.

Cinnamon: Cinnamon is a fragrant spice often used in both sweet and savory dishes. It is rich in antioxidants and has anti-inflammatory properties. Cinnamon can help regulate blood sugar levels, reduce heart disease risk, and improve brain function. Sprinkle cinnamon on oatmeal, yogurt, or add it to baked goods and curries for a warm, comforting flavor.

Cayenne Pepper: Cayenne pepper is a spicy addition to many dishes and offers numerous health benefits. It contains capsaicin, a compound known for its metabolism-boosting properties and ability to reduce pain. Cayenne pepper can also help improve circulation and support digestive health. Add a pinch of cayenne pepper to soups, stews, and marinades for an extra kick.

Incorporating Herbs and Spices into Your Diet

Experiment with Recipes: Try new recipes that incorporate a variety of herbs and spices to discover new flavors and health benefits.

Use Fresh and Dried Herbs: Both fresh and dried herbs can be used to enhance your dishes. Fresh herbs add a burst of flavor, while dried herbs are convenient and can be used year-round.

Make Herbal Teas: Herbal teas are a simple and delicious way to enjoy the benefits of herbs. Try brewing teas with ginger, turmeric, or cinnamon for a soothing and healthful beverage.

By adding these traditional herbs and spices to your meals, you can enjoy a diverse range of flavors while reaping their nutritional benefits. It is a simple and tasty way to boost your health and well-being.

 Navigating nutrition for frail adults does not have to be complex. With careful planning, a touch of creativity, and respect for cultural food preferences, meals can become a foundation of resilience and joy in the later years. By focusing on nutrient-dense foods, experimenting with flavors, and appreciating traditional dishes, we can enhance health, happiness, and the overall quality of life. So, let us celebrate the journey of eating well with every meal, making nutrition a key component of thriving in the golden years.

CHAPTER 8: FUTURE OF NUTRITION AND FRAILTY RESEARCH

As we venture into the future, the intersection of nutrition and frailty research is buzzing with innovation. Picture a world where your meal plan is as unique as your fingerprint, where gadgets not only count your steps but also monitor your nutrient intake, and where your DNA holds the secrets to your dietary needs. Let us embark on this journey through the crystal ball of nutrition science.

8.1 Innovations In Personalized Nutrition For Frailty

Imagine walking into a café, and instead of the usual menu, you are handed a dish crafted specifically for your body's needs. Sounds like science fiction? Welcome to the era of personalized nutrition! This approach tailors dietary recommendations to individual characteristics, aiming to enhance health outcomes, especially in managing frailty among older adults.

Recent studies highlight the potential of personalized nutrition strategies. For instance, a study published in 'The Lancet' investigated the use of personalized nutrition to help patients meet protein and caloric goals, reducing the risk of adverse clinical outcomes (72). By considering factors like genetics, lifestyle, and health status, personalized nutrition can address specific nutritional deficiencies and support muscle strength, necessary for frailty prevention.

Moreover, the InCluSilver project (Innovation in personalised Nutrition through Cluster cooperation in the Silver economy) emphasizes innovations in personalized nutrition for older adults, including wearable devices that monitor health and lifestyle, providing data to customize dietary plans (73). The project has successfully generated 37 new products and services focused on personalized nutrition for older adults, addressing their unique dietary needs and preferences. One example is a chocolate bar with lemon balm designed to help older adults fall asleep more easily. This integration of technology and nutrition science paves the way for more effective frailty management strategies.

8.2 Technology In Monitoring And Improving Nutrition

Gone are the days when keeping a food diary meant scribbling in a notebook. Today, technology has revolutionized how we monitor and improve our nutrition, playing a pivotal role in managing frailty.

Mobile health interventions, like the 'Olitor' app, have shown promise in promoting healthier eating habits among older adults with frailty. The Olitor app is a mobile application designed to help older adults eat healthier and adhere to a Mediterranean diet. Developed by Master of Science in Information Management (MSIM) students at the University of Washington in collaboration with the University of Washington School of Nursing, the app is particularly aimed at older adults, including those with dementia or mild cognitive impairments. A pilot study revealed that such interventions could improve adherence to the Mediterranean diet, increase the intake of recommended foods, and potentially enhance overall health outcomes (74).

Additionally, self-monitoring tools empower older adults to make informed dietary decisions. Nutrition apps provide valuable health-related information, facilitating patient-centered care and potentially improving frailty outcomes (74). These apps can help users track their dietary habits, plan balanced meals, and receive personalized nutrition advice, all of which contribute to better health management. By using these apps, individuals can gain insights into their nutritional intake, identify areas for improvement, and make informed dietary choices. The integration of artificial intelligence in these tools can offer personalized feedback, further enhancing their effectiveness.

Key Benefits of Nutrition Apps

Personalized Nutrition Plans: Many nutrition apps offer customized meal plans and recommendations based on individual health conditions, dietary preferences, and goals. This personalized approach ensures that users receive advice tailored to their specific needs, enhancing the effectiveness of their nutritional strategies.

Diet Tracking: Users can log their daily food intake, monitor calorie consumption, and keep track of essential nutrients like vitamins and minerals. This tracking capability helps individuals stay accountable and make adjustments to their diet as needed.

Educational Resources: Nutrition apps often include educational content, such as articles, videos, and tips on healthy eating. This information empowers users with the knowledge they need to make healthier choices and understand the impact of nutrition on their overall well-being.

Health Monitoring: Some apps integrate with wearable devices and health monitoring tools, allowing users to track their physical activity, sleep patterns, and other health metrics alongside their diet. This holistic approach provides a comprehensive view of one's health.

Community Support: Many apps have social features that allow users to connect with others, share experiences, and seek support from a community of like-minded individuals. This sense of community can motivate users to stay on track with their health goals.

Improving Frailty Outcomes

Nutrition apps can play a significant role in addressing frailty, especially in older adults. Frailty is often associated with poor nutritional status, and targeted nutritional interventions can help mitigate its effects. By providing tailored dietary advice and tracking nutritional intake, nutrition apps can support the following:

Enhanced Nutrient Intake: Ensuring that individuals consume adequate amounts of essential nutrients can improve overall health and vitality, reducing the risk of frailty.

Weight Management: Maintaining a healthy weight is essential in preventing frailty. Nutrition apps can help users achieve and maintain their ideal weight through balanced meal plans and portion control.

Improved Muscle Strength: Protein intake is vital for muscle health. Apps can guide users on how to incorporate sufficient protein into their diet, helping to maintain muscle mass and strength.

Better Digestive Health: By promoting the consumption of fiber-rich foods and probiotics, nutrition apps can support gut health, which is linked to overall well-being and resilience.

In summary, nutrition apps provide valuable tools and information that facilitate patient-centered care, enabling individuals to take control of their health and potentially improve outcomes related to frailty. By leveraging technology, users can access personalized nutrition guidance, track their progress, and make informed decisions to support their overall well-being.

8.3 Advances In Nutritional Genomics

Ever wondered why your friend thrives on a high-carb diet while you feel sluggish just looking at a bagel? The answer might lie in your genes. Nutritional genomics or Nutrigenomics, the study of how our genes interact with our diet, is shedding light on these mysteries.

Research indicates that genomic instability may help anticipate frailty in older adults, suggesting that understanding an individual's genetic makeup can inform targeted nutritional interventions to improve frailty outcomes (75). By tailoring nutrition plans based on genetic profiles, we can potentially delay the onset of frailty and enhance quality of life.

How Nutrigenomics Works

Nutrigenomics combines the study of nutrition, genomics, and molecular biology to understand how our diet interacts with our genes. By analyzing an individual's genetic makeup, we can identify specific genetic variations that influence how they metabolize nutrients, respond to certain foods, and their risk for diet-related conditions like diabetes, obesity, and cardiovascular diseases (76).

Benefits of Personalized Nutrition:

Prevention and Management of Chronic Diseases: Customized diets can help prevent and manage conditions like diabetes mellitus, heart disease, and obesity by addressing individual risk factors and metabolic profiles.

Enhanced Weight Management: Personalized nutrition plans consider factors such as metabolism and hormone levels, making weight loss or gain more effective and sustainable.

Improved Mental Health: Diet plays a critical role in mental health. Personalized nutrition can help alleviate symptoms of depression and anxiety by addressing specific nutrient deficiencies.

Optimized Athletic Performance: Athletes benefit from personalized nutrition by receiving diets that enhance performance and recovery based on their unique physiological needs.

Impact on Frailty

Frailty is often linked to poor nutritional status, and targeted nutritional interventions can help mitigate its effects (77). By ensuring adequate nutrient intake and maintaining muscle strength, personalized nutrition can reduce the risk of frailty and improve overall well-being.

In summary, by tailoring nutrition plans based on genetic profiles, we can create highly individualized dietary recommendations that optimize health outcomes, delay the onset of frailty, and enhance the quality of life. This approach represents a transformative shift in dietary science, moving away from one-size-fits-all diets to personalized nutrition strategies that cater to individual needs (78). Furthermore, advances in nutrigenomics research elucidate the synergistic roles of genetics and nutrition in health, paving the way for precision nutrition approaches that consider individual genetic variations (79). This personalized approach holds promise for more effective frailty management strategies.

8.4 Policy To Combat Frailty Through Nutrition

The Power of Policy-Level Interventions

While individual choices are crucial for maintaining health, the collective power of policy-level interventions should not be overlooked. These interventions can create environments that promote healthy aging and combat frailty through improved nutrition.

Comprehensive Frailty Management Strategies

Implementing comprehensive frailty management strategies, including nutritional support, exercise programs, and fall prevention strategies, can significantly impact public health (8). These strategies include:

Nutritional Support: Ensuring older adults have access to nutritious foods tailored to their dietary needs can help maintain their health and prevent frailty.

Exercise Programs: Regular physical activity is essential for maintaining muscle strength and mobility. Community-based exercise programs can encourage older adults to stay active.

Fall Prevention: Developing and promoting fall prevention strategies can reduce the risk of injuries and improve overall safety for older adults.

Supportive Policies

Policies that support access to nutritious foods, provide education on healthy eating, and promote active lifestyles are essential in addressing the multifactorial nature of frailty. These policies can include:

Food Access Programs: Initiatives like community gardens, farmers' markets, and food assistance programs can make nutritious foods more accessible to older adults.

Educational Campaigns: Public health campaigns that educate older adults about the importance of a balanced diet and regular exercise can encourage healthier choices.

Active Living Initiatives: Policies that promote physical activity, such as building safe walking paths and providing community fitness classes, can support active lifestyles.

Integrating Technology

Integrating technology into public health initiatives can enhance the effectiveness of nutrition programs. For example:

AI-Enabled Smart Speakers: Using in-home, AI-enabled smart speakers to deliver personalized nutrition information and health management advice can reduce access barriers and support healthy aging. These devices can provide tailored meal plans, reminders for medication and appointments, and even connect users with healthcare professionals for virtual consultations (80, 81).

Health Apps and Wearables: Mobile health apps and wearable devices can track dietary intake, physical activity, and vital signs, providing valuable data for personalized health management. These technologies can help older adults monitor their health and stay on track with their wellness goals.

The Future of Nutrition and Frailty Research

The future of nutrition and frailty research is a dynamic tapestry woven with personalized approaches, technological advancements, genetic insights, and supportive policies. By embracing these innovations, we can empower individuals to age with strength and resilience, transforming the twilight years into a golden era of vitality.

In conclusion, combining individual efforts with policy-level interventions and technological innovations can create a comprehensive approach to healthy aging. By working together, we can build supportive environments that promote well-being and combat frailty, ensuring a better quality of life for older adults.

ABBREVIATIONS

AI: Artificial Intelligence

ATP: Adenosine Triphosphate

BMD: Bone Mineral Density

CFS: Clinical Frailty Scale

CVD: Cardiovascular Disease

DM: Diabetes mellitus

DNA: Deoxyribonucleic Acid

EFS: Edmonton Frail Scale

FFP: Fried Frailty Phenotype

FI: Frailty Index

FRAIL: Fatigue, Resistance, Ambulation, Illnesses, and Loss of Weight

GFI: Groningen Frailty Indicator

InCluSilver: Innovation in Personalised Nutrition through Cluster Cooperation in the Silver

ISAR: Identification of Seniors at Risk

MNA: Mini Nutritional Assessment

MSIM: Master of Science in Information Management

MUST: Malnutrition Universal Screening Tool

MVP: Most Valuable Player

PT: Physical Therapist

SCFA: Short-Chain Fatty Acids

SHARE-FI: Survey of Health, Ageing and Retirement in Europe-Frailty Instrument

TFI: Tilburg Frailty Indicator

TLC: Tender Loving Care

TUG: Timed Up and Go

USPSTF: United States Preventive Services Task Force

UV: Ultraviolet

VIP: Very Important Person

REFERENCES

1. Fried LP, Tangen CM, Walston J, Newman AB, Hirsch C, Gottdiener J, et al. Frailty in Older Adults: Evidence for a Phenotype. The Journals of Gerontology: Series A. 2001; 56 (3): M146-M57.

2. Rockwood K, Mitnitski A. Frailty defined by deficit accumulation and geriatric medicine defined by frailty. Clin Geriatr Med. 2011; 27 (1): 17-26.

3. Rockwood K, Song X, MacKnight C, Bergman H, Hogan DB, McDowell I. A global clinical measure of fitness and frailty in elderly people. Can Med Assoc J. 2005; 173 (5): 489-95.

4. Rockwood K, Theou O. Using the Clinical Frailty Scale in Allocating Scarce Health Care Resources. Can Geriatr J. 2020; 23 (3): 210-5.

5. Dent E, Kowal P, Hoogendijk EO. Frailty measurement in research and clinical practice: A review. European Journal of Internal Medicine. 2016; 31: 3-10.

6. O'Caoimh R, Sezgin D, O'Donovan MR, Molloy DW, Clegg A, Rockwood K, et al. Prevalence of frailty in 62 countries across the world: a systematic review and meta-analysis of population-level studies. Age and Ageing. 2020; 50 (1): 96-104.

7. Toson B, Edney LC, Haji Ali Afzali H, Visvanathan R, Khadka J, Karnon J. Economic burden of frailty in older adults accessing community-based aged care services in Australia. Geriatrics & Gerontology International. 2024; 24 (9): 939-47.

8. Angulo J, El Assar M, Álvarez-Bustos A, Rodríguez-Mañas L. Physical activity and exercise: Strategies to manage frailty. Redox Biol. 2020; 35: 101513.

9. Moraes MBd, Avgerinou C, Fukushima FB, Vidal EIO. Nutritional interventions for the management of frailty in older adults: systematic review and meta-analysis of randomized clinical trials. Nutrition Reviews. 2020; 79 (8): 889-913.

10. Woo J, Goggins W, Sham A, Ho SC. Social determinants of frailty. Gerontology. 2005; 51 (6): 402-8.

11. Pilotto A, Ferrucci L, Franceschi M, D'Ambrosio LP, Scarcelli C, Cascavilla L, et al. Development and Validation of a Multidimensional Prognostic Index for One-Year Mortality from Comprehensive Geriatric Assessment in Hospitalized Older Patients. Rejuvenation Research. 2008; 11 (1): 151-61.

12. Fried LP, Cohen AA, Xue QL, Walston J, Bandeen-Roche K, Varadhan R. The physical frailty syndrome as a transition from homeostatic symphony to cacophony. Nat Aging. 2021; 1 (1): 36-46.

13. Ghosh TS, Rampelli S, Jeffery IB, Santoro A, Neto M, Capri M, et al. Mediterranean diet intervention alters the gut microbiome in older people reducing frailty and improving health status: the NU-AGE 1-year dietary intervention across five European countries. Gut. 2020; 69 (7): 1218-28.

14. Lorenzo-López L, Maseda A, de Labra C, Regueiro-Folgueira L, Rodríguez-Villamil JL, Millán-Calenti JC. Nutritional determinants of frailty in older adults: A systematic review. BMC Geriatrics. 2017; 17 (1): 108.

15. Shirley Chao, Judy Simon, Laura Borth, Lydia McGrath, Jaime Gahche, Mary Beth Arensberg, et al. 2024; Pages Accessed at American Society of Aging at on 29 December 2024.

16. Buhl SF, Beck AM, Olsen PØ, Kock G, Christensen B, Wegner M, et al. Relationship between physical frailty, nutritional risk factors and protein intake in community-dwelling older adults. Clinical Nutrition ESPEN. 2022; 49: 449-58.

17. Chen X, Zhang Z, Yang H, Qiu P, Wang H, Wang F, et al. Consumption of ultra-processed foods and health outcomes: a systematic review of epidemiological studies. Nutr J. 2020; 19 (1): 86.

18. Zupo R, Donghia R, Castellana F, Bortone I, De Nucci S, Sila A, et al. Ultra-processed food consumption and nutritional frailty in older age. Geroscience. 2023; 45 (4): 2229-43.

19. Piggott DA, Tuddenham S. The gut microbiome and frailty. Transl Res. 2020; 221: 23-43.

20. Halfon M, Phan O, Teta D. Vitamin D: a review on its effects on muscle strength, the risk of fall, and frailty. Biomed Res Int. 2015; 2015: 953241.

21. Guo Y, Miao X, Hu J, Chen L, Chen Y, Zhao K, et al. Summary of best evidence for prevention and management of frailty. Age and Ageing. 2024; 53 (2).

22. Lagoumintzis G, Patrinos GP. Triangulating nutrigenomics, metabolomics and microbiomics toward personalized nutrition and healthy living. Human Genomics. 2023; 17 (1): 109.

23. Yeung SSY, Kwan M, Woo J. Healthy Diet for Healthy Aging. Nutrients. 2021; 13 (12).

24. Tapsell LC, Neale EP, Probst Y. Dietary Patterns and Cardiovascular Disease: Insights and Challenges for Considering Food Groups and Nutrient Sources. Curr Atheroscler Rep. 2019; 21 (3): 9.

25. Scarmeas N, Stern Y, Tang MX, Mayeux R, Luchsinger JA. Mediterranean diet and risk for Alzheimer's disease. Ann Neurol. 2006; 59 (6): 912-21.

26. Moore DR. Keeping Older Muscle "Young" through Dietary Protein and Physical Activity. Advances in Nutrition. 2014; 5 (5): 599S-607S.

27. Wilkinson DJ, Piasecki M, Atherton PJ. The age-related loss of skeletal muscle mass and function: Measurement and physiology of muscle fibre atrophy and muscle fibre loss in humans. Ageing Research Reviews. 2018; 47: 123-32.

28. Moore DR, Churchward-Venne TA, Witard O, Breen L, Burd NA, Tipton KD, et al. Protein ingestion to stimulate myofibrillar protein synthesis requires greater relative protein intakes in healthy older versus younger men. J Gerontol A Biol Sci Med Sci. 2015; 70 (1): 57-62.

29. Soysal P, Isik AT, Carvalho AF, Fernandes BS, Solmi M, Schofield P, et al. Oxidative stress and frailty: A systematic review and synthesis of the best evidence. Maturitas. 2017; 99: 66-72.

30. Qin B, Panickar KS, Anderson RA. Cinnamon: potential role in the prevention of insulin resistance, metabolic syndrome, and type 2 diabetes. J Diabetes Sci Technol. 2010; 4 (3): 685-93.

31. Peng Y, Ao M, Dong B, Jiang Y, Yu L, Chen Z, et al. Anti-Inflammatory Effects of Curcumin

in the Inflammatory Diseases: Status, Limitations and Countermeasures. Drug Des Devel Ther. 2021; 15: 4503-25.

32. Riehl L, Fürst J, Kress M, Rykalo N. The importance of the gut microbiome and its signals for a healthy nervous system and the multifaceted mechanisms of neuropsychiatric disorders. Frontiers in Neuroscience. 2024; 17.

33. Di Napoli A, Pasquini L, Visconti E, Vaccaro M, Rossi-Espagnet MC, Napolitano A. Gut-brain axis and neuroplasticity in health and disease: a systematic review. La radiologia medica. 2024.

34. Sandoval-Insausti H, Pérez-Tasigchana RF, López-García E, García-Esquinas E, Rodríguez-Artalejo F, Guallar-Castillón P. Macronutrients Intake and Incident Frailty in Older Adults: A Prospective Cohort Study. J Gerontol A Biol Sci Med Sci. 2016; 71 (10): 1329-34.

35. Chuy V, Gentreau M, Artero S, Berticat C, Rigalleau V, Pérès K, et al. Simple Carbohydrate Intake and Higher Risk for Physical Frailty Over 15 Years in Community-Dwelling Older Adults. J Gerontol A Biol Sci Med Sci. 2022; 77 (1): 10-8.

36. Tanaka T, Kafyra M, Jin Y, Chia CW, Dedoussis GV, Talegawkar SA, et al. Quality Specific Associations of Carbohydrate Consumption and Frailty Index. Nutrients. 2022; 14 (23).

37. Zhang H, Wei X, Pan J, Chen X, Sun X. Anemia and frailty in the aging population: implications of dietary fiber intake (findings of the US NHANES from 2007–2018). BMC Geriatrics. 2023; 23 (1): 634.

38. Gómez-Pinilla F. Brain foods: the effects of nutrients on brain function. Nat Rev Neurosci. 2008; 9 (7): 568-78.

39. Sandoval-Insausti H, Pérez-Tasigchana RF, López-García E, García-Esquinas E, Rodríguez-Artalejo F, Guallar-Castillón P. Macronutrients Intake and Incident Frailty in Older Adults: A Prospective Cohort Study. The Journals of Gerontology: Series A. 2016; 71 (10): 1329-34.

40. Tomata Y, Wang Y, Hägg S, Jylhävä J. Fatty Acids and Frailty: A Mendelian Randomization Study. Nutrients. 2021; 13 (10): 3539.

41. Shen JX, Lu Y, Meng W, Yu L, Wang JK. Exploring causality between bone mineral density and frailty: A bidirectional Mendelian randomization study. PLoS One. 2024; 19 (1):

e0296867.

42. Ogawa M, Sato Y, Nagano F, Yoshimura Y, Kuzuya M. Mineral supplementation in patients with frailty and sarcopenia-a systematic review. Geriatr Gerontol Int. 2024; 24 (9): 850-8.

43. Tan BL, Norhaizan ME, Liew WP, Sulaiman Rahman H. Antioxidant and Oxidative Stress: A Mutual Interplay in Age-Related Diseases. Front Pharmacol. 2018; 9: 1162.

44. El Assar M, Angulo J, Rodríguez-Mañas L. Frailty as a phenotypic manifestation of underlying oxidative stress. Free Radical Biology and Medicine. 2020; 149: 72-7.

45. Liu L, Wu X, Zhang B, Yang W, Li D, Dong Y, et al. Protective effects of tea polyphenols on exhaustive exercise-induced fatigue, inflammation and tissue damage. Food Nutr Res. 2017; 61 (1): 1333390.

46. Liu Y-J, Zhan J, Liu X-L, Wang Y, Ji J, He Q-Q. Dietary flavonoids intake and risk of type 2 diabetes: A meta-analysis of prospective cohort studies. Clinical Nutrition. 2014; 33 (1): 59-63.

47. Shrime MG, Bauer SR, McDonald AC, Chowdhury NH, Coltart CEM, Ding EL. Flavonoid-Rich Cocoa Consumption Affects Multiple Cardiovascular Risk Factors in a Meta-Analysis of Short-Term Studies[1]. The Journal of Nutrition. 2011; 141 (11): 1982-8.

48. ter Borg S, Verlaan S, Hemsworth J, Mijnarends DM, Schols JM, Luiking YC, et al. Micronutrient intakes and potential inadequacies of community-dwelling older adults: a systematic review. Br J Nutr. 2015; 113 (8): 1195-206.

49. Xu Y, Liu X, Liu X, Chen D, Wang M, Jiang X, et al. The Roles of the Gut Microbiota and Chronic Low-Grade Inflammation in Older Adults With Frailty. Frontiers in Cellular and Infection Microbiology. 2021; 11.

50. Belobrajdic D, Brownlee I, Hendrie G, Rebuli M, Bird T. Gut health and weight loss: An overview of the scientific evidence of the benefits of dietary fibre during weight loss. CSIRO, Australia; 2018.

51. Singh RK, Chang H-W, Yan D, Lee KM, Ucmak D, Wong K, et al. Influence of diet on the gut microbiome and implications for human health. Journal of Translational Medicine. 2017; 15 (1): 73.

52. Lim MY, Nam YD. Gut microbiome in healthy aging versus those associated with frailty. Gut Microbes. 2023; 15 (2): 2278225.

53. Diakité MT, Diakité B, Koné A, Balam S, Fofana D, Diallo D, et al. Relationships between gut microbiota, red meat consumption and colorectal cancer. J Carcinog Mutagen. 2022; 13 (3).

54. Lee C, Lee J, Eor JY, Kwak MJ, Huh CS, Kim Y. Effect of Consumption of Animal Products on the Gut Microbiome Composition and Gut Health. Food Sci Anim Resour. 2023; 43 (5): 723-50.

55. Besora-Moreno M, Llauradó E, Valls RM, Pedret A, Solà R. Effects of Probiotics, Prebiotics, and Synbiotics on Sarcopenia Parameters in Older Adults: A Systematic Review and Meta-Analysis of Randomized Controlled Trials. Nutrition Reviews. 2024.

56. Sánchez YSdlBB, Martínez Carrillo BE, Aguirre Garrido JF, Martínez Méndez R, Benítez Arciniega AD, Valdés Ramos R, et al. Emerging Evidence on the Use of Probiotics and Prebiotics to Improve the Gut Microbiota of Older Adults with Frailty Syndrome: A Narrative Review. J Nutr Health Aging. 2022; 26 (10): 926-35.

57. Ni Lochlainn M, Bowyer RCE, Moll JM, García MP, Wadge S, Baleanu A-F, et al. Effect of gut microbiome modulation on muscle function and cognition: the PROMOTe randomised controlled trial. Nature Communications. 2024; 15 (1): 1859.

58. Loh JS, Mak WQ, Tan LKS, Ng CX, Chan HH, Yeow SH, et al. Microbiota–gut–brain axis and its therapeutic applications in neurodegenerative diseases. Signal Transduction and Targeted Therapy. 2024; 9 (1): 37.

59. Park KJ, Gao Y. Gut-brain axis and neurodegeneration: mechanisms and therapeutic potentials. Frontiers in Neuroscience. 2024; 18.

60. Zheng Y, Bonfili L, Wei T, Eleuteri AM. Understanding the Gut–Brain Axis and Its Therapeutic Implications for Neurodegenerative Disorders. Nutrients. 2023; 15 (21): 4631.

61. Siripaopradit Y, Chatsirisakul O, Ariyapaisalkul T, Sereemaspun A. Exploring the gut-brain axis in alzheimer's disease treatment via probiotics: evidence from animal studies-a systematic review and meta-analysis. BMC Neurology. 2024;24(1):481.

62. Kate W. 2024; Pages: https://www.care.com/c/quick-easy-healthy-meals-for-seniors/ on 29 December 2024.

63. National Council of Aging 2024; Pages: https://www.ncoa.org/article/5-tips-for-seniors-creating-healthy-meal-plans/ on 29 December 2024.

64. John S. 2024; Pages: https:// taking.care/blogs/resources-advice/ultimate-guide-to-meal-prepping-for-seniors/ on 29 December 2024.

65. Tripp F. The Use of Dietary Supplements in the Elderly: Current Issues and Recommendations. Journal of the American Dietetic Association. 1997; 97 (10): S181-S3.

66. Yan L-C, Yu F, Wang X-Y, Yuan P, Xiao G, Cheng Q-Q, et al. The effect of dietary supplements on frailty in older persons: a meta-analysis and systematic review of randomized controlled trials. Food Science and Technology. 2022; 42.

67. U.S. Preventive Services Task Force 2024; Pages Accessed at 29 December at https://www.uspreventiveservicestaskforce.org/uspstf/draft-recommendation/ vitamin-d-calcium-combined-supplementation-primary-prevention-falls-fractures-communitydwelling-adults 2024.

68. America SSO; Pages: https: //seniorservicesofamerica.com/blog/loss-of-appetite-in-elderly/ on 29 December 2024.

69. Pilgrim AL, Robinson SM, Sayer AA, Roberts HC. An overview of appetite decline in older people. Nurs Older People. 2015; 27 (5): 29-35.

70. Paula G. Harris-Swiatko, Wendy J. Dahl 2024; Pages: https://edis.ifas.ufl.edu/publication/FS214Paula G. Harris-Swiatko and Wendy J. Dahl on 29 December 2024.

71. Satia JA. Diet-related disparities: understanding the problem and accelerating solutions. J Am Diet Assoc. 2009; 109 (4): 610-5.

72. Schuetz P, Fehr R, Baechli V, Geiser M, Deiss M, Gomes F, et al. Individualised nutritional support in medical inpatients at nutritional risk: a randomised clinical trial. Lancet. 2019; 39 3(10188): 2312-21.

73. Burton DGA, Wilmot C, Griffiths HR. Personalising nutrition for older adults: The InCluSilver project. Nutrition Bulletin. 2018; 43 (4): 442-55.

74. Ni Lochlainn M, Cox NJ, Wilson T, Hayhoe RPG, Ramsay SE, Granic A, et al. Nutrition and Frailty: Opportunities for Prevention and Treatment. Nutrients. 2021; 13 (7).

75. Sánchez-Flores M, Marcos-Pérez D, Lorenzo-López L, Maseda A, Millán-Calenti JC, Bonassi S, et al. Frailty Syndrome and Genomic Instability in Older Adults: Suitability of the Cytome Micronucleus Assay As a Diagnostic Tool. The Journals of Gerontology: Series A. 2018; 73 (7): 864-72.

76. Heather Yoshimura 2024; Pages: https://www.rupahealth.com/post/personalized-nutrition-tailoring-diet-plans-to-genetic-profiles?form=MG0AV3 on 31 December 2024.

77. Ni Lochlainn M, Cox NJ, Wilson T, Hayhoe RPG, Ramsay SE, Granic A, et al. Nutrition and Frailty: Opportunities for Prevention and Treatment. Nutrients. 2021; 13 (7): 2349.

78. Singar S, Nagpal R, Arjmandi BH, Akhavan NS. Personalized Nutrition: Tailoring Dietary Recommendations through Genetic Insights. Nutrients. 2024; 16 (16): 2673.

79. Cole JB, Gabbianelli R. Editorial: Recent advances in nutrigenomics: Making strides towards precision nutrition. Front Genet. 2022; 13: 997266.

80. Faltaous S, Janzon S, Heger R, Strauss M, Golkar P, Viefhaus M, et al. Wisdom of the IoT Crowd: Envisioning a Smart Home-based Nutritional Intake Monitoring System. Proceedings of Mensch und Computer 2021. Ingolstadt, Germany: Association for Computing Machinery; 2021: 568–73.

81. Michel M, Burbidge A. Nutrition in the digital age - How digital tools can help to solve the personalized nutrition conundrum. Trends in Food Science & Technology. 2019; 90: 194-200.